WHAT READERS ARE SAYING ABOUT
YOUR BEAUTIFUL BODY

This book has helped me get back into my skinny jeans! As the mother of three young children, I never imagined that I could lose the weight that I had accumulated over the years, and actually look leaner and more toned that ever. I have lost 9 ½ inches so far! I am getting so many compliments now!

❖ Denise Hanono

Lariesa is truly someone that has dedicated her life to teaching others the importance of living a fit and healthy lifestyle. Her passion and determination for health, fitness, and wellness has made Lariesa one of the foremost Pilates and fitness professionals in the country.

❖ Alan Harris
founder/creator of Absolute Body Power Media

The tips in the book have helped me lose 10 inches, and shed fat. I am the type of person who doesn't like to work out, so I was amazed that I have been able to stick with it, and see such great results! The best part is that I am too busy to devote a lot of time to exercise, so I needed something that was quick and effective. This book gave me just the motivation and encouragement that I needed!

❖ Ana Corona

YOUR BEAUTIFUL BODY

Using Pilates to Overcome Your Weight Loss Obstacles

By
Lariesa Bernick ACE, BBU

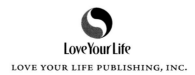
LOVE YOUR LIFE PUBLISHING, INC.

All rights reserved. No part of this book may be used or reproduced in any manner whatsoever without written permission except in the case of brief quotations embodied in articles and reviews.

Notice: Please consult with your personal physician prior to beginning any diet or exercise plan. The information in this book is intended to supplement the advice of your personal physician, whom you should consult about weight concerns and any medical conditions you may have.

Love Your Life Publishing, Inc
7127 Mexico Road Suite 121
Saint Peters, MO 63376
www.LoveYourLifePublishing.com
publisher@LoveYourLifePublishing.com
1-800-314-5590

ISBN: 978-1-934509-35-7
Library of Congress Control Number: 2010936609

Cover Design by: www.MonkeyCMedia.com
Internal Design: www.Cyanotype.ca
Additional typesetting: www.masterpagedesign.co.uk

First Printing: 2011
Printed in China

ACKNOWLEDGEMENTS

I would like to thank the following people for their participation in the success of this book:

Christine Messier, Your Voice, Inc. – Collaborative Editor
Jennifer Thompson – Monkey C Media, cover photo and design
Denise Conrad- Denise C Photography, Interior photography
Kenneth Montiel- Cover photo makeup
Laura R. Otero- exercise section model
ToeSox- sponsor

For their professional support and training:

Alan Harris - Absolute Body Power
Lizbeth Garcia- Tilcia Studios
My brother, Marcus- for his technical expertise, love, and patience
Manuel Saenz- for the never ending love, support, and encouragement

And to my parents, for teaching me that I can accomplish anything I put my mind to! I love you both.

Dedication

To my parents who have made everything possible for me, and to my son who inspires me to be the best person I can be.

TABLE OF CONTENTS

Preface	i
Introduction	iii
CHAPTER ONE: *The Power of Pilates*	1
The benefits of Pilates	1
Key principles of the Pilates method	2
Benefits of regular physical activity	4
CHAPTER TWO: *Overcoming Common Weight Loss Obstacles*	7
If you don't feel comfortable in the gym	7
Even the thought of exercising makes you tired	8
When you feel you just cannot find the time	9
When you lack motivation	11
When exercise becomes boring	13
The other side of the coin - cardio	14
Your health: expense or investment?	15
Strategies for budget-conscious workouts	17
Moderation- slow and steady...	18
CHAPTER THREE: *Pilates at Home – Tools and Strategies*	21
Key elements to making exercise effective	21
Illustrated exercise programs	23

CHAPTER FOUR: *Pilates for Rehabilitation and Prevention of Back Pain*   55

What causes back pain?   55

Pilates helps correct posture   57

Pilates develops core strength   60

Pilates promotes flexibility   61

Considerations for back pain patients   61

Pilates has a way of making simple exercises effective   62

Avoiding loaded flexion   62

Tips for decreasing back pain   63

Key elements to making your workout effective   64

CHAPTER FIVE: *Anti-Aging Strategies for a Lean and Beautiful Body*   67

Your metabolism   67

Eat your way to beautiful skin   71

Take supplements as an insurance policy for your health   72

Eat foods rich with fiber   74

Water is your fountain of youth   77

Limit your consumption of sweets and salty snacks   78

Consume alcohol in moderation   80

CHAPTER SIX: *D.I.E.T.: Divine Inspiration for Everyday Triumphs*   83

Positive diet acronyms   83

Budgeting calories   85

Calculating Resting Metabolic Rate (RMR)   87

Calculating daily calories burned for weight loss   88

CHAPTER SEVEN: *The Food Factor*   93

What *do* I eat?   93

What *should* I eat?   94

Meal ideas   95

Healthy substitutions   100

Not-so-innocent snacking   101

Sneaky sources of sugar   102

Beverages make a huge difference	103
Stress and Anxiety	104
Making small changes	105
Strategies for long-term success	107
Hidden saboteurs	108
I eat really healthy and I exercise but I am not losing weight!	109
Beware of high-fat condiments and foods	109
It's impossible to eat right at work!	110
How can I avoid sabotaging myself at a restaurant?	111
The carbohydrate controversy	112
The Power of Protein	115
CHAPTER EIGHT: *Lareisa's Favorite Healthy Recipes*	119
About the Author	133

PREFACE

I have always loved the finesse and power of the human body. I love learning about it and my passion is sharing that knowledge with my clients. My career began as an Aerobics Instructor because I really enjoyed the energy and dynamic moves of an aerobics class. What I felt I was missing from my contribution was the one-on-one connection with my clients. When I decided to expand into personal training I also became interested in the strength and core movements of Pilates and grew my business by working with people in their homes as a certified Pilates instructor and personal trainer.

I did all of the training myself, and three years later I had too many clients to continue to travel to their homes so I turned my garage into a little Pilates studio with one reformer. The demand for Pilates and personal training with the type of care and personal commitment I was providing drew into more clients than there were hours in the day. My clients all had their individual goals and needs for working out and I honored that with personalized sessions that not only worked on weight loss, but strength and recovery. Some clients were healthy and wanted to lose weight and tone up, while others included young women with crippling rheumatoid arthritis, older adults with degenerative disc disease, sciatica, and scoliosis, and the list goes on. I had the passion and drive to work with all of these individuals, creating mobile healthy bodies and minds.

Even though there were never enough hours in the day, there was always a desire to work with even more people. Within nine months Pilates of Eastlake opened its doors. I wanted to give everyone the opportunity to reach their goals and change their bodies and minds, all within a wide range of price options, and not a single membership fee. It was my best attempt to meet and touch countless more people's lives and bodies. Six months after opening, we have five certified instructors, and we work with hundreds of clients each week. This is just the beginning for Pilates of Eastlake, and for my journey in leading people to results.

INTRODUCTION

Let's face it, there are many weight loss and core strength tricks, fads and gimmicks on the market. And why do we fall for them? Because we want something quick, inexpensive and somewhat effortless that will solve our problems. Whether you want to lose weight, successfully recover from surgery or an accident, or just be stronger and healthier, you can do it with the help of simple, consistent strategies and tools that will change the way you feel about your body and your life.

This book is for anyone who has struggled to find physical relief and emotional strength in what sometimes feels like a never-ending battle to be healthy. If you are like me, you have been excited about a new plan or a new resolve and then something holds you back. You want to find an exercise system that you enjoy doing, but you don't want it to become routine and boring. You want the diversity of different exercises but you don't want to join a gym. You want to strengthen your body but at the same time you don't want to have chronic joint or muscle pain. You want to reduce fat but you don't want to spend every morning or evening working out. I hear you. I am right there with you and I can help.

Let's spend a little bit of time addressing the issues around exercise and the journeys that people have shared with me and then let's make the changes together. Allow me to show you some of the strategies I have learned along the way, not only from my experience, but also from my clients. The best way to avoid pitfalls and struggles and to increase your chance of success is to have the knowledge of what others have gone through to achieve success. There is no reason to reinvent the wheel when you can expedite the learning process by matching the techniques used by others. You might just find that you share their goals and can overcome the same obstacles. Read on to see what they are, and how you can learn how they overcame them.

Disclaimer: Stories provided in this book are real however the names have been changed to respect the privacy of the individual. The author does not claim to be a medical or nutritional professional. The recommendations and exercises are intended to be used in conjunction with a healthy diet and under the supervision of a physician.

CHAPTER ONE

THE POWER OF PILATES

"A few well-designed movements, properly performed in a balanced sequence, are worth hours of doing sloppy calisthenics or forced contortion."

❧ JOSEPH PILATES

Pilates dramatically transforms the way your body looks, feels, and performs. It is said that Pilates works the body from "the inside out." It focuses on creating a sleek and toned physique that is mobile and healthy. It slenderizes the thighs and flattens the abdomen. It teaches body awareness, good posture, flexibility and agility. It also relieves back pain by strengthening the core and the muscles that support the spine. Imagine being lean, strong, and free from back pain at any age! Looking younger and healthier in the process doesn't hurt either. This is the beauty of Pilates.

The Benefits of Pilates

- ❧ Builds strength and lean muscles
- ❧ Increases flexibility, mobility and coordination
- ❧ Develops core strength and control
- ❧ Improves body control and awareness
- ❧ Enhances maximum efficiency of organ function
- ❧ Promotes relaxation, balance and focus
- ❧ Increases endurance
- ❧ Creates flat abdominals and defined muscles
- ❧ Provides a safe and effective workout without strain and impact

Pilates exercises are so gentle to your body and yet gives it a challenging workout. This makes it a popular way to get into shape. It can also be used for physical therapy or rehabilitation exercises.

Pilates develops a strong "core", or center of the body. The core consists of your abdominals, back, and pelvic area. Since you do not move your arms and legs without the assistance of your core, strengthening this area can affect everything you do. You can create lean muscles that are flexible and able to move with control and a healthy range of motion. It creates a balanced strength within the body that allows you to be very mobile.

You will learn how to condition your whole body in an evenly balanced and conditioned way. This helps you to enjoy daily activities, and enhance sports performance. During Pilates exercises, no muscle group is over- or under-trained. In conventional workouts, it is common to create stronger areas and muscle groups, leading to muscular imbalance which is the primary cause of injury and chronic back pain. Pilates trains several muscle groups at once, in smooth continuous movements. It trains the body to work in a safe and efficient manner that is valuable for injury recovery, sports performance, good posture, and optimal health.

Pilates is unique in that it enhances the mind-body connection by emphasizing breathing, correct spinal, shoulder, and pelvis alignment, and by concentrating on smooth flowing movement. The control and efficiency of the motion trains the body to become very aware and effective in the way that it moves. Of course, proper breathing reduces stress and lets the muscles move effectively.

KEY PRINCIPLES OF THE PILATES METHOD OF MOVEMENT:

1. **Concentration:** Be present with your mind and body. Concentrate on the way your body is moving so that you are making the most of your exercise time. When you concentrate on how an exercise feels

THE POWER OF PILATES   3

while you are doing it, you will get more out of the exercise, and you will feel it working more effectively. It is far more effective and safe to do fewer repetitions with the correct movement than twice as many with an incorrect form.

2. **Breathing**: Use the rhythm of your breath to maintain the connection between mind and body. Oxygenation is what helps to keep the body healthy and revitalizes your entire body with clean air. Breathing deeply expels stale air from the depths of your lungs and cleanses the bloodstream through oxygenation. The fresh air will energize your mind and your muscles. Through these full deep breaths you also improve your lung capacity.

3. **Control**: Joseph Pilates' philosophies originated with this concept of controlling your muscles throughout the entire exercise to make the most of the movements. In other words, it is extremely important not to rush or go through the exercises in a sloppy careless way. This would lead to injury and a lack of solid results. To produce the best results, each motion must be done with control and purpose, slowly and with precision.

4. **Centering**: All Pilates' movements start with the core or "powerhouse." The powerhouse consists of the large muscle groups in our center which encompass our abdomen, lower back, hips, and buttocks. Every movement that you do with your arms and legs originates from your center. A golfer cannot swing his arm without a strong center, for example. This is true even in our daily lives and tasks such as reaching down to lift a bag of groceries. A strong core is the foundation for strong and healthy movement. Developing this center helps to build a body structure that will be the foundation for good health.

5. **Precision**: Precision is the end result of concentration, control and centering. This comes only from practice and its rewards are the creation of core strength and optimum vitality. Every movement in

Pilates has a purpose. Each detail is important to achieve maximum results. Focus on doing a single precise and perfect movement rather than several halfhearted ones.

6. **Fluidity:** Pilates exercises are not made up of isolated movements. There is a sense of rhythm and flow that creates graceful, smooth movement patterns. There are no jerky, quick, or forceful motions in Pilates. It is about moving with grace and control, in an energetic and dynamic way.

7. **Harmony and Relaxation:** When Pilates exercises are done with ease and flow it creates a sense of rejuvenation after the workout, rather than exhaustion. Listen to your body when you are going through each movement. Do not force movements if it feels unnatural. If something doesn't feel right or causes pain, then stop! In time you will be able to feel the effectiveness of the exercises as you perform them, and this will lead to the results that you are looking for.

BENEFITS OF REGULAR PHYSICAL ACTIVITY:

1. **Exercise improves your mood.** After a stressful day, a 30-minute workout is just what you need to focus and relax. Exercise stimulates chemicals in the brain which leave you feeling happier and more relaxed than you were before you worked out! Your self-esteem will also get a boost when you look and feel better. Exercise not only improves your mood and outlook on life, it also reduces feelings of anxiety.

2. **Exercise lowers your risk for chronic diseases:**

❖ **High blood pressure:** Regular aerobic activities can lower blood pressure.

THE POWER OF PILATES

- **Cigarette smoking:** Smokers who become physically active are more likely to cut down or stop smoking.

- **Diabetes:** People at their ideal weight are less likely to develop diabetes. Physical activity may also decrease insulin requirements for people with diabetes.

- **Obesity and overweight:** Regular physical activity can help people lose excess fat or stay at a reasonable weight.

- **High levels of triglycerides:** Physical activity helps reduce triglyceride levels. High triglycerides are linked to developing coronary artery disease in some people.

- **Low levels of HDL:** Low levels of HDL ("good") cholesterol (less than 40 mg/dL for men/less than 50 mg/dL for women) have been linked to a higher risk of coronary artery disease. Recent studies show that regular physical activity can significantly increase HDL cholesterol levels and thus reduce your risk.

3. **If you really want to lose weight, you need to exercise!** Exercise causes the body to burn calories, and the more intense the workout, the more calories you burn. This will allow you to maintain or even lose weight. Remember, when it comes to maintaining weight think "calories in = calories out". If you eat more calories than you burn, you will gain weight. But the opposite is also true. You do not need to set aside major time to work out! Just take the stairs at work instead of the elevator. Or take a brisk walk on your lunch break. Do jumping jacks during the commercials. Put your TV by your treadmill, and do not allow yourself to watch your favorite show unless you are walking while you watch! These extra daily activities will add up to calories burned, and pounds at bay!

4. **Exercise gives you more energy.** Exercise delivers oxygen and nutrients to your tissues, and causes the blood to circulate through your heart and blood vessels. Your heart and lungs will work more efficiently

which will provide you with more energy to do the things that you enjoy!

5. **Exercise helps you sleep at night.** It is recommended to get at least 8 hours of shut-eye every night for the body to function properly. A good night's sleep can improve your concentration, productivity and mood. If you aren't able to fall asleep, or have a difficult time staying asleep, you may need to do more physical activity. Since exercising boosts your heart rate and increases circulation, it will also wake you up and give you energy, so avoid working out within two hours of your bedtime. Otherwise you may find that you can't fall asleep!

    I have a pet peeve about getting enough sleep. It truly gives me the energy and clarity I need to get through my day. It also prevents me from getting sick, and keeps my skin looking good. As a single mother, this is no easy task! I make it a priority to go to bed early (right after my son it seems), and try to get through my own exercise early in the day.

6. **A sizzling sex life.** If you aren't in the mood for sex, or are too tired or out of shape for physical intimacy, regular exercise can help. It leaves you feeling energized, happier, and more confident. Even inconsistent exercise can boost the way you feel about yourself, and put you more in the mood. It also improves your circulation which can lead to more satisfying sex. According to the Mayo Clinic, men who exercise are less likely to have problems with erectile dysfunction than are men who don't exercise, especially as they get older.

7. **Practice seeing exercise as a special time for YOU to do something good for yourself!** You may treat yourself to a day at the spa to feel pampered, but why not put exercise on that list? If you practice viewing exercise as a time for you to do something wonderful for your body, you will be more likely to want to do it. Make exercise fun! Forget about dragging yourself to the elliptical if you hate it; instead get outside in the sunshine for a walk with your dog, or play with your kids at the park.

CHAPTER TWO

OVERCOMING COMMON WEIGHT LOSS OBSTACLES

"If you can find a path with not obstacles, it probably doesn't lead anywhere."

❖ FRANK A. CLARK

Now that we have explored the benefits of exercise, let's address what has been holding us back. Yes, we ARE going to overcome your objections - together. I am not saying I have heard all of the excuses, but I can tell you I have heard a lot.

IF YOU DON'T FEEL COMFORTABLE IN THE GYM

First of all, you are not the only one who feels this way. In fact, I would say that the majority of people would rather not have to work out in the fitness club setting. Sarah came to me feeling guilty that she hadn't been exercising because she felt intimidated to work out at her local gym. She didn't have the right clothes, or the right body to feel like she fit in. She wasn't comfortable being there. I hear this every day, and I assured Sarah that she was not alone. If you feel intimidated by your local gym environment, then you aren't very likely to want to go! The good news is that there are other options that are just as effective.

Strategies for gym-phobia

- If you are brave enough to workout at your local gym, then give yourself credit for being there to make your body healthy and fit! That's why you're there after all: to make a commitment to lifelong fitness.

- Ask a friend to meet you or start talking to other people who are already members who tend to work out around the same time you do. Knowing you have a buddy will not only provide you with the sense of accountability to work out, but you will also not feel alone in your efforts to show up in your most comfortable clothes, with no make-up on and your hair pulled back.

- Workout on your own at home. This book will give you all of the tools to get you started on the right track. By the time you begin to get more fit, your self-confidence will improve, and you may become more comfortable to go to the gym. Or you may decide that in-home fitness is perfect for you!

EVEN THE THOUGHT OF EXERCISING MAKES YOU TIRED

Maybe you feel too tired and lazy to even consider getting up for a jog. You need to set yourself up for success in a way that will work for *you*.

Strategies for the inactive

- Setting realistic expectations is the first thing to consider. If you feel like you need to start exercising everyday and eating better, then you may never start. That seems like a pretty big hurdle if you are just starting out. Rather, praise yourself for doing the tiniest activity, such as walking for 10 minutes after dinner. If you start by doing this a couple of times per week then those 10 minutes will eventually turn into 15 minutes, or you might add on another day. Starting with baby steps is the key to making it work, and DO not expect to do more. Congratulate yourself for small steps, and I promise they will turn into larger ones. If you start with too much too early, then you set yourself up for failure.

❖ Don't work against yourself! If I thought I had to work out at 4pm every day, then I would fail before I started. At 4pm, I am much more interested in taking a nap than exercising. I know that it is my low-energy time of day. I'm a morning person, so exercising while I have the energy to do so and am still motivated works better for me. Maybe you have more energy in the evening. That may be a better time for you to get active.

❖ Set an appointment to exercise. It is almost impossible to feel like you have time to exercise, so pencil it in to your schedule (or better yet, use a pen!), and don't let anything else get in the way. It is not abnormal to have to carve out a spot in your busy schedule to make exercise happen.

❖ Carry workout clothes, a bottle of water, and tennis shoes in your car. If you are prepared, it is more likely to happen. If you work out first thing in the morning, then lay your shoes and clothes out the night before where you will trip over them (not quite that literally) so that you feel guilty not putting them on.

WHEN YOU FEEL YOU JUST CANNOT FIND THE TIME

My father always told me that there are two things we will always need more of: time and money. As it turns out, he was right. The older I get, the more of these commodities I need. The trouble is that I never seem to have enough of either, and probably never will. We will talk about the money issue in a moment, so for now, let's talk time. Let's face it there will never be enough time in the day to get everything done and your workout too. But wait! Don't think this is the excuse to not work out. It isn't. You just have to get creative.

John came limping into my studio late one afternoon. He was a good looking man, only in his forties, but acting as though he were in his eighties. He had a lot of pain and stiffness associated with a sedentary lifestyle. He had never been into fitness during his young life, and his busy executive job didn't give him the time to exercise. Now that his life was being affected, John wanted me to fix him. The sad news is that he is too young to feel so old, but the good news is that he is not too old to have the health and fitness that he desired. Although he still works his busy job, he is now making time for exercise. He spends less than one hour a week in my studio with me, and the rest of the time doing exercise at home. This program has worked so well for him that I can hardly keep up with his progress each time he comes to see me. So the question is, "how does John fit exercise into his busy schedule?" He did it the same way that you will, by getting creative at sneaking it in wherever there are opportunities, and by eliminating activities that just aren't as important.

Strategies for the time-starved

- Go for a brisk 15-minute walk on your lunch break. No excuses. It has been proven that several shorter bursts of exercise throughout the day offer similar benefits as one long workout.

- You've heard it before: park farther away from your destination so that you can walk quickly from the car. Remember, a couple of walks to and from the car at this distance can add up!

- TiVo your favorite show to watch later. Get active now! I know it sounds painful, but you'll get over it. It won't hurt as much as losing your health with age, trust me.

- Get up 15 minutes earlier to walk on the treadmill. Do not fill in this time with something else!

- Do a few exercises as outlined in this book while you're watching TV. Commit to this three times per week, and plan it around specific shows and times.

- Walk or jog down the sidewalk, and take your kids with you. You'll burn fat while they get quality time with you.

- Maybe you need to become a weekend warrior. Those lazy Saturday mornings can turn into a refreshing walk with a friend or your kids. The weekends just might be your chance to get moving!

WHEN YOU LACK MOTIVATION

I asked Gina why she never missed a Pilates class or personal training session with me. I knew it couldn't be because I was that much fun to hang out with. So I asked her what it was that kept her coming back and committed. If only we could all be so enlightened! As it turns out, Gina was not motivated to come to class just because she dreamt of a smaller waist size, or because she had a class reunion to prepare for. No, her driving force was much more mundane than that, and much more achievable on a daily basis. She got her workouts in because it made her feel better the moment she was done. Instant gratification! She even admitted not wanting to get out of bed to exercise on several occasions, but she usually made it because she reminded herself how great she would feel afterward. So how can you use this to help yourself gain a little motivation? Let me ask you this: what motivates you to get up and make coffee every morning? Ahhh... because you know it will give you the kick you need to get through your morning.

Let's look at some motivating reasons to exercise that don't have anything to do with losing weight:

- Sense of accomplishment

- Mood boost

- Better outlook on life

- Higher self-esteem

- Increase in productivity

- Decrease in healthcare costs

- Looking and feeling younger

- Lowering your risk for heart disease, diabetes, high blood pressure, and so much more!

Here is what some of my clients have shared with me:

- *"The end result: I feel good when I finish my workout."* - Anonymous

- *"The knowledge that what I do for my body makes a major difference in how I feel and look. That goes for "good" and "bad" food also!"* - Nona, 73 years old

- *"I want to lose this pregnancy weight quickly!"* - Elizabeth, 31 years old

- *"I want to be healthy, stay strong, and be HAPPY from the inside."* - Chinda

- *"Appearance!"* - Jill, 45 years old

- *"I feel more centered and less stressed when I workout. It makes me feel good about my day knowing that I did something healthy for myself."* - Betsy, 29 years old

- *"I am motivated by feeling good, having energy, and creating toned muscles".* - Cheryl, 60 years old

- *"I feel better physically and mentally."* – Anonymous

- *"My friends motivate me to exercise! They help to make the process more fun."* - Carmen, 38 years old

- *"I love how strong my body feels, especially during a workout!"* - Missy, 41 years old

- *"I have three kids, and my weight fluctuates a lot. I am motivated to maintain a healthy weight. It makes me feels good all around. Your metabolism slows down as you age, and I want to stay healthy!"* - Sally, 37 years old

- *"I am motivated to exercise so that I feel better, look better, and live longer."* - Kathy, 43 years old

- *"My family encourages me to exercise so that I will not get sick. I want to have a long and healthy life, and my family encourages me to do something about it."* - Reena

- *"I want to maintain balance in my life. Exercise allows me to indulge in all of life's gifts without guilt!"* - Laura, 32 years old

WHEN EXERCISE BECOMES BORING

Exercise can become boring, especially when you are doing something repetitive day after day. Of course, it takes a certain amount of discipline to be fit, and you can't expect it to be overly-exciting to stay in the same exercise routine. The feeling of accomplishment and added energy should help to motivate you to get out and exercise.

Strategies to prevent boredom with your exercise routine.

- Think of it as a treat for yourself. It's your time for yourself or with your friends, away from the kids, away from the stresses of work, while giving you the opportunity to take care of your body. How do you feel when you get a manicure? Like you are doing something special for yourself to be pretty, right? Well there you go. It's mind over matter.

- Don't do the exact same workout day after day. Try cycling, walking, swimming, golfing, or a local salsa dancing class! Exercise can be anything that gets you moving, and variety will get you results faster by working more muscle groups in different ways.

- Team up with a friend or a walking group from work for a great way to create a supportive environment that can help to keep you accountable.

THE OTHER SIDE OF THE COIN - CARDIO

A lot of people ask me what they should do outside of Pilates or strength training to help them reach their fitness goals. What is my answer? Cardio of course! I know you didn't want to hear that, but you already know it's true. The best possible scenario to get into shape is by combining 2-3 days of strength conditioning and toning such as Pilates, with a few days of cardio (aerobic exercise).

Cardiovascular activity is any exercise that boosts your heart rate and gets your lungs working. It can be as simple as going for a brisk walk or swimming. It doesn't matter if you do longer, less frequent sessions of aerobic exercise, or shorter, more frequent sessions. You may also do three 10-minute bursts of exercise for aerobic benefit. The important thing is that you do it!

For healthy adults younger than age 65, the American Heart Association and the American College of Sports Medicine recommend at least 30 minutes of moderate intensity activity most days of the week. Moderate intensity activity boosts your heart rate to 50-85% of your maximum heart rate. So how do you determine your ideal exercising heart rate?

Subtract your age from 220 (226 for women) to get your approximate maximum heart rate. For example, if you are a 50-year-old woman wishing to find your target heart rate, then you would subtract 50 from 226 which would give you 176. You should exercise at a heart rate that is about 70 % of this, or about 123 beats per minute. More importantly, however, is to feel like you are getting a good workout.

The Rate of Perceived Exertion indicates that it is best to feel like you are getting a challenging workout. It is not even necessary to monitor your heart rate as long as you feel challenged. In other words, if you feel like you're slacking off on the intensity, then you are! On a scale of 1-10, where 10 is the most possible effort, and 1 is resting, then you should be exercising at an intensity of about 7. See? No need for fancy heart rate monitors.

My rule of thumb: if you are able to carry on a conversation easily with someone while you are working out, then you are not working hard enough. You should barely be able to carry on a broken conversation.

YOUR HEALTH:
EXPENSE OR INVESTMENT?

Is there anything you would hide from your own husband or significant other in an attempt to lose weight? Women are especially good at putting in the extra miles when it comes to their beauty and weight loss efforts. Unfortunately, these miles seldom come in the form of distance on the treadmill. Dania comes to Pilates classes regularly. She doesn't like sweating in a big gym or feeling like she has to wear certain clothes, or look a specific way. So she chooses to do her workout in our small studio setting. She appreciates the workout which leaves her feeling great, and an atmosphere that isn't intimidating. I am convinced that she would move into my studio if she could. Her diligence has paid off: several inches lost, and a smaller-sized new wardrobe to prove it.

However, Dania has made it very clear that I am not to tell her husband how much she pays to attend her regular Pilates classes and private training sessions. I don't know how I got in the middle of this! In fact, she goes out of her way to save just enough money from her monthly budget to continue her workout program because she loves the way she feels and looks. I give her credit for giving her body-sculpting Pilates sessions so much priority in her life, and still maneuvering around her financial obstacles. Just please leave me out of it!

And then there is Janet who has had a gym membership for years now. She pays monthly for the membership and for all of the promises that it is suppose to give her. Unfortunately, Janet doesn't even go to the gym. She pays her monthly dues each month but does not reap any benefit from her membership. The problem is that Janet doesn't know what other options exist to help her reach her goals, without setting foot into the gym. In fact, 40% of my clients have a gym membership that they never use. Another 30% don't have a membership at all. That leaves only 30% that actually have and use theirs. So why are you spending that money for something that doesn't serve you? Just because you pay for the service doesn't mean that it will magically get you in the door! Do yourself a favor: let it expire. Save yourself the money and find a Plan B that will actually work for you. Let's find some better options for you!

Now, I don't suggest starting an exercise program by delegating finances to where they don't belong, but I do suggest coming up with a plan that will work for you personally. The issue of deciding how much is necessary to pay for training, gym memberships, etc. is personal, and must be calculated into a budget. So how much must a person pay to get the body they want? Of course there are a lot of factors involved, such as physical limitations and financial flexibility, but in general goals can be reached without spending any money. I promise. Whether your goal is to lose weight and tone up, or become free from pain, there are a lot of options for you. These options include expensive ways such as hiring a personal trainer, and less expensive ways such as getting a gym membership, or working out at home. Surprisingly, I have been working with people in their home for years without fancy equipment, and they have been just as successful as those with expensive gym memberships. So what can you do on your own that will produce results?

Strategies for budget-conscious workouts

- Do strengthening exercises at home. Exercise bands are very inexpensive, and are just as effective as using weights. You can tone up the entire body with a resistance band, and its light enough to go with you when you travel.

- Start a walking group by placing an ad on Craigslist or encourage your friends to join you instead of hitting Happy Hour. Everybody wants and needs support to exercise!

- Try an exercise video. Amazon.com offers great prices, or you can even check them out at your local library.

- Take the stairs, or park your car farther away from your destination.

- Sign up for an aerobics class at your local community center or recreation department. These can be an affordable way to stay in shape and learn something new! You might find a workout buddy there or even be able to get the kids involved with a community project while you're getting fit!

- Check out smaller, private studios that offer fun and effective programs. These studios have a homey atmosphere with support from people with similar goals in a non-intimidating environment. You are also more likely to get results with their individual support.

- Find individual cost effective classes that will keep you financially accountable.

- Look online for private groups that meet in local parks, such as Meetup.com

- Talk with neighbors or co-workers who you can walk with for support and accountability.

MODERATION – SLOW AND STEADY...

Red flags go up in my mind when someone comes to me to start an exercise program and they are excited to work out every day. It tells me right away that they won't be at it for long. Tammy was just such a client. She was determined to start her exercise program (which happened to be a New Year's resolution) off on the right foot by exercising every day and watching what she ate. I advised against such a busy start, but she couldn't understand my reasoning. So she went off on her own to reach her goals in record time. A few months later she was back in my studio, having not only fallen off the wagon, but also gaining back more weight than she had started with. Tammy was eager to learn a way that would work for her and make her results permanent. That way is called limitation.

Losing weight is 50% action and 50% psychological strength. The trick is to come up with a plan that you won't mind sticking to. Not too much anyway. Start slow with tiny changes then add more small changes as the first ones become permanent. If you rush through the stages, you will fail. The longer you take to incorporate these adjustments into your lifestyle, the more likely they are to stick. Rushing through the stages is where psychological strength comes in. Recognize the feeling of wanting to do too much too fast, and limit yourself to only slow steps. For example, you may feel up to exercising five days a week during the second week into your new workout plan, but don't. Only allow yourself to do two days that week. Stick to it and your plan will succeed. Physically fit people have learned how to make diet and exercise a part of their daily life, not just for this month or this year. Learn to moderate your diet and activity changes to grow into your life. Remember this is a *lifestyle* change for life so there is no need to rush it.

SCHEDULE FOR OPTIMUM RESULTS:

Week 1 & 2	Do cardio such as walking or jogging for 30 minutes 2 times per week
Week 3 & 4	Increase cardio time to 30-40 minutes and frequency to 3 times per week
Week 5 & 6	Continue the same as Week 4 and add one 1-hour Pilates or strength training day
Week 7 & 8	Continue the same as Week 4 and add two 1-hour Pilates or strength training days
Third Month	Repeat Week 8 and increase cardio to 40 minutes and 4 days per week
Fourth Month	Turn cardio into intervals of a slow pace for 3 minutes, fast pace for 2 minutes. Keep cardio to 40 minutes and 3 days per week and two 1-hour Pilates or strength training days.

CHAPTER THREE

PILATES AT HOME — TOOLS AND STRATEGIES

"Physical fitness is not only one of the most important keys to a healthy body, it is the basis of dynamic and creative intellectual activity."

❖ JOHN FITZGERALD KENNEDY

KEY ELEMENTS TO MAKING EXERCISE EFFECTIVE

There are a few details that will help you achieve the most results from your at-home mat Pilates workouts. The proper positioning of the body and mental awareness all play a role in the effectiveness of your workout. In Pilates, the right conditions include a balance of strength, flexibility, symmetry, alignment, and good, stable posture.

1. The Main Focus

In traditional workouts, we have been taught to think about the body in terms of the arms, legs and torso. Movements that involved the legs created a focus in that area. Now we must change our focus to the torso, and everything that surrounds it. Everything you do with the arms and legs originates from your torso, or midsection, which is also called the powerhouse. This is true even in the smallest of tasks. You cannot reach up to get something from the shelf, or take the dog for a walk without involving your torso. This area consists of everything between the neck and top of the legs. It contains the vertebral column and the major organs. Remember that each movement comes from this area, which stabilizes the body and assists in every movement.

2. The Powerhouse

The powerhouse describes all the muscles that circle the midsection of the body. That includes the abdominals, lower back, hips, and buttocks. When these areas are under-toned, it can cause lower back pain and discomfort. Lack of strength and mobility in this area also leads to the bloated "gut" and "muffin top" areas that can be difficult to combat. Not with Pilates! Everything we do in Pilates helps to strengthen and tone this area. You must be aware of using good posture and correct form in the exercises (and all the time!). Lengthen the torso, pull your shoulders down and back, and engage your abdominals. Your posture will protect your lower back and will make your workouts more effective.

3. Scooping Your Belly In

Have you noticed that if your back arches your belly pooches out? This is common, and creates weak abdominal muscles, a pooched out tummy, and a tight back. This posture makes the muscles build outwardly, away from the spinal column. Training the muscles this way makes it very difficult to support the lumbar region of the back, or to create a lean waistline (See Figure I). Instead, learn to maintain a posture that scoops in the belly and lengthens the back. This is called "scooping the belly" or "pulling your naval to your spine". This position lets you use your abdominal muscles to reinforce the Paraspinal muscles (they run alongside your spine to support it). The action strengthens these muscles, allowing it to be strong and mobile. It also allows the abdominals to be able to contract and engage —very important if you want to flatten and tone your belly. (See Figure II)

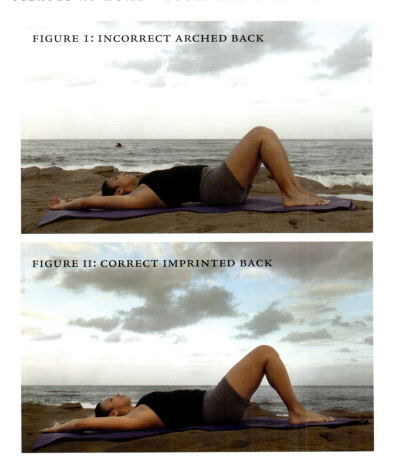

FIGURE I: INCORRECT ARCHED BACK

FIGURE II: CORRECT IMPRINTED BACK

Ok, now that you know what "scooping the belly" does for you, let's talk about how to make that happen. First, it is *not* about sucking your stomach in and consequently holding your breath. Instead, think about anchoring your belly button in towards your spine. When you are lying on a mat, gently tilt your pelvis so that your pubic bone lifts, and your lower back makes gentle contact with the mat. Try this exercise: exhale forcefully and feel what happens to your belly. Your abdominals pull in and your core muscles engage. Now hold that flexed feeling without changing your breathing. This does become easier with practice!

4. Balanced Muscle Integration

Performing movements in Pilates requires you to think about the entire body as a whole, balanced unit. It has been common practice to isolate a particular muscle group by focusing on them when they are in motion. The problem with this ideology is that it ignores the muscles groups that are not moving, creating an unbalanced body. This is partly why Pilates is so effective; you never neglect any part of the body during any exercise. The body becomes strong everywhere in a balanced and dynamic way. Even the smallest muscle groups are integrated into every movement. How can we accomplish this thorough, full-body focus in each exercise? It is best to think of "anchoring" or "stabilizing" the part of the body that is not in motion. For example, if you are lying on your back and doing single leg circles, then you will focus on stabilizing the torso and hips while the leg moves in a controlled manner. In other words, don't let the hips rock and roll around as the leg moves. Anchor your hips and shoulders onto the mat and keep them stable throughout the motion of the leg. Moving in this way will utilize all of the muscles of your powerhouse or core, and will help to flatten and tone the abdominals, strengthen the back, and your legs. You see, doing the motion correctly by using your entire body in a balanced way will produce the most effective results.

5. Lower Body Stabilization

Stabilizing the body is an important way to engage all of the muscle groups while performing any exercise. It allows the muscles to work effectively while avoiding injury. Another area to focus on stabilizing is the lower body. If you are doing an abdominal or upper body exercise, you would not want the legs to be moving or flailing about. To create a stable lower body, engage the legs by squeezing the back of the upper inner thighs. The toes will point out slightly in a V-shape as you squeeze your legs and gluteus, almost as though you were zipping up your inner thighs. Do not lock your knees or become rigid. This position is meant to engage the muscles in a soft, supporting way. And voila! You are now working and toning your thighs as you perform the exercise.

6. Muscle Control Without Tension

One of the reasons Pilates can be an enjoyable strain-free workout is because you are engaging and challenging the muscles without tensing or straining. With other exercises, we have become accustomed to tensing up, holding our breath, and pushing to the point of strain in order to reach our goals. We actually want to accomplish the opposite effect to truly move effectively and safely. The movements require strength and concentration, and there is a natural rhythm and flow to the motion. Moving with the breath can help you to accomplish this. Breathe in a natural way, inhaling at the beginning of a movement, and exhaling throughout its completion. If you find you are holding your breath, you may be working at a level that is too intense, or you may be tensing the muscles as you perform the movement. Make sure you are working at the proper level for your body, relax and engage your muscles, and breathe. If you finish your workout by feeling that your muscles were challenged, but there was no stress or strain, then you have learned to control your muscles without tension!

The rest of this chapter will focus on more exercises that you can do at home to help you tone up and lose weight. Using Toesox is an option that may help you feel more secure on the mat during your workout. These exercises all have emphasis on strengthening your core muscles, which is what you need to tighten and strengthen your midsection. Start with the Beginning section, which is demonstrated by Laura Otero, and do the exercises in order. Then progress to the Intermediate/Advanced section, demonstrated by myself, as soon as you are ready for a greater challenge. All of the exercises must be done with control and effort. It is possible to go through them quickly and mindlessly, which would be pointless. Remember, this is your workout, so make it count! Focus on moving with strength and breathe throughout the motion, making each movement precise. The sequence of exercises in each section should not take more than 30 minutes, and I recommend doing them at least twice per week. You should have more energy, be less stressed, and see your waistline shrink in a few short weeks. Don't forget that you will also have a strong, mobile, and healthy back. This is your time!

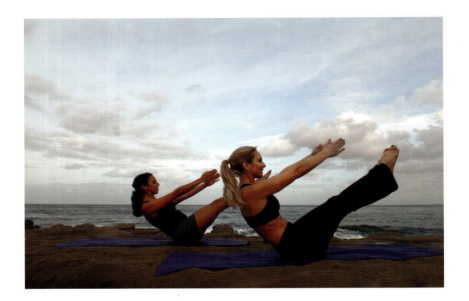

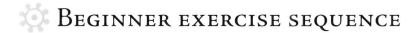

Beginner exercise sequence

The proper back position for the exercises:

Lie on your back and move the hips to create a hollow between your back and the mat. This is called an anterior pelvic tilt. Avoid this position while doing the exercises, as it could put excess strain on the lower back.

To work the abdominals effectively and place the body in a safe position, tilt the pelvis so that the lower back makes gently contact with the mat. This is a posterior pelvic tilt (or an imprint), and will ensure maximum results. Now, keep this position… and here we go!

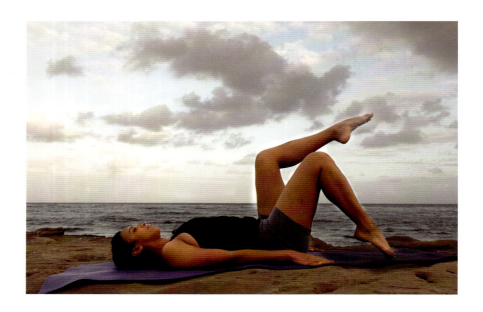

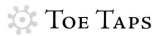 TOE TAPS

1. Lie on your back with knees up at a 90 degree angle and your lower leg parallel to the floor.
2. Inhale, feel the pressure on your lower back and pelvis.
3. Exhale; tap one toe to the floor without letting the lower back arch up off the mat. Engage your abdominals.
4. Focus on keeping the torso perfectly still as the legs move.

Purpose: to strengthen the abs and back.
Reps: 10 times, then repeat

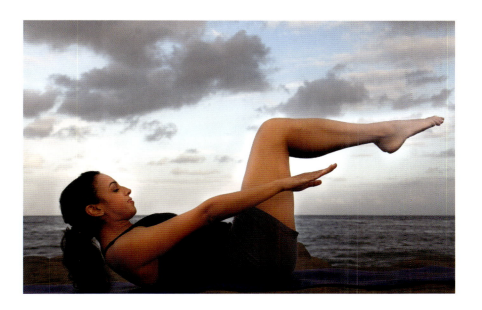

☼ Hundred Preps

1. Lie on your back with your arms at your sides, knees bent and your feet flat on the floor.
2. Inhale; reach your arms to the ceiling while keeping your back on the mat, ribs pulled in.
3. Exhale, lower the arms and roll the head and shoulders off the mat. Gently pulse the arms by your sides.
4. Inhale for 5 pulses of the arms, and exhale for 5, working up to a total of 100.

Purpose: to strengthen abs

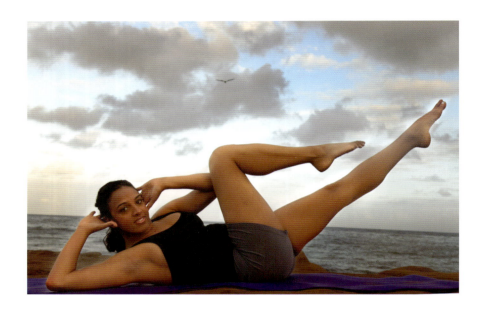

☼ Modified Criss Cross

1. Lie on your back with your arms by your sides and your legs in a 90 degree angle.
2. Keep your back touching the mat and your abs engaged as you move the legs as though riding a bicycle.
3. Exhale every time the leg extends. Feel the torso stabilize through the motion.

Purpose: to strengthen abs.
Reps: 10 times then repeat

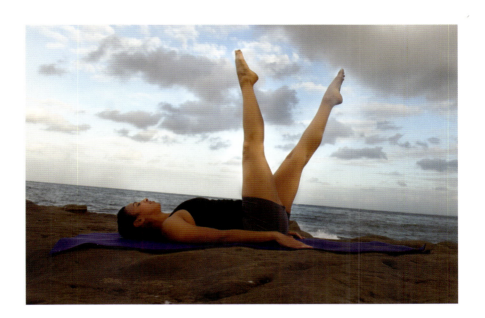

☀ Scissors Kicks

1. Lie on your back with your arms by your sides and your legs straight up.
2. Pull your abs in and remember your imprint!
3. Exhale as you slowly kick the legs like scissors, with control. Feel your abs engage with each kick. Make the kicks only as large as you can while keeping the back on the mat, pelvis stable.

Purpose: Strengthen the abs and back.
Reps: 10-20 kicks

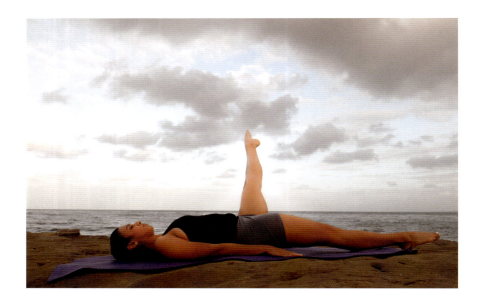

☀ Single Leg Circles

1. Lie on your back with one leg stretched out, pressing the heel into the floor. The other leg is pointed straight up to the ceiling, relax your hands beside you.
2. Exhale as the leg circles around the outside, and inhale as it returns to the top.
3. Keep the motion in control without moving the pelvis. Repeat on both legs.

Purpose: to strengthen the abs, increase hip flexibility and pelvic stability.
Reps: 15 circles on each leg

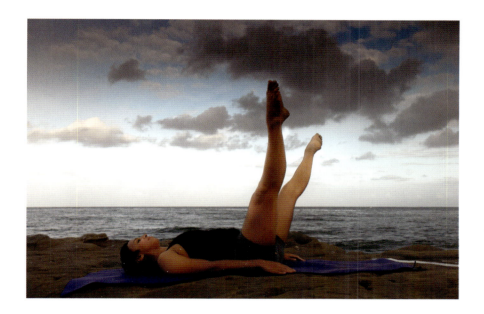

☼ Open/Close Legs

1. Lie on your back with your arms by your sides and your legs straight up.
2. Pull your abs in and imprint the spine.
3. Inhale as you open the legs, exhale and close the legs.
4. Don't let your legs drop towards the floor unless you are able to maintain contact on the mat with your back (your imprint). The stronger the abs are, the lower you are able to drop the legs without losing your imprint!

Purpose: Strengthen the abs and back, and to create a stable pelvis
Reps: 10 kicks, then repeat

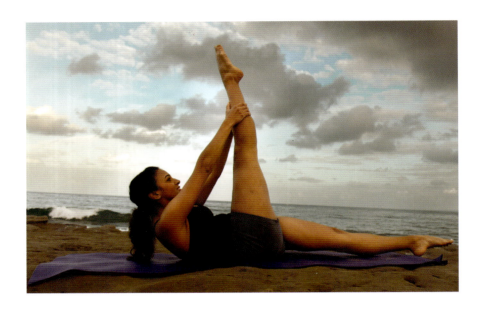

✹ Single Straight Leg Stretch

1. Lie on your back with the head and shoulders lifted off the mat, legs straight up towards the ceiling.
2. Gently pull one leg towards you as the other lowers. Do not lower the leg any farther than you can maintain a stable pelvis. No rocking and rolling around!
3. Exhale each time you catch a leg; alternate.

Purpose: to strengthen the abs, flexibility of the hamstrings
Reps: 10 each side

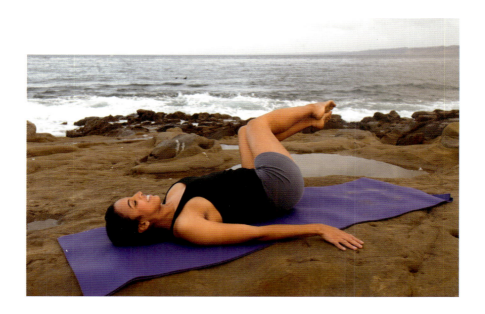

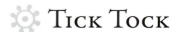 ## Tick Tock

1. Lie on your back with your legs at 90 degrees and your arms on the floor away from your sides.
2. Exhale as you drop both knees to one side while keeping the opposite shoulder on the floor. Inhale and drop the knees to the other side.
3. Do not let the knees rest on the floor.

Purpose: to stretch back and sides, increase the mobility of the spine.
Reps: 10

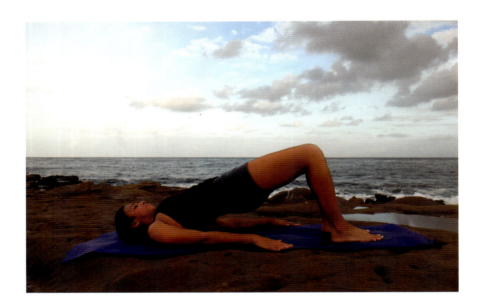

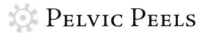 PELVIC PEELS

1. Lie on your back with your feet on the floor hip distance apart, and your arms beside you.
2. Exhale, tilt your pelvis off the floor and roll your hip up towards the ceiling, one vertebra at a time. Roll back down, pressing the spine into the floor one vertebra at a time. Pretend that the spine is a string of pearls.

Purpose: to strengthen the back and legs, mobility of the spine
Reps: 10

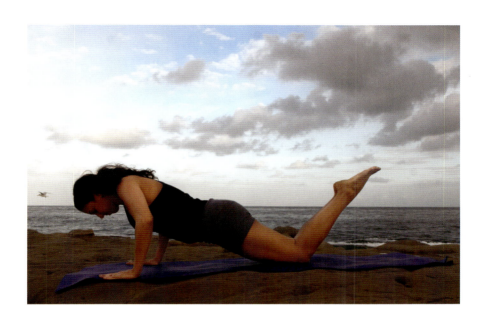

✸ Modified Push Ups

1. Begin in an all-fours position, hands wide.
2. Stretch out one leg behind you. Lower the chest and hips towards the floor as though you were a flat board. Pull your belly in; exhale and lower.

Purpose: To strengthen the upper body
Reps: 8-10 pushups, then switch legs and repeat

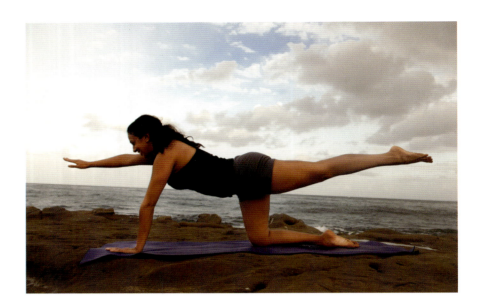

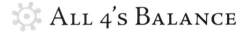 ## All 4's Balance

1. Begin on all fours, with your belly pulled in and limbs square.
2. Exhale as you extend one leg out and opposite arm. Balance in this position, eventually working up to adding little pulses of the arm and leg. Do all on one side before switching.

Purpose: to strengthen the back
Reps: hold for 30 seconds

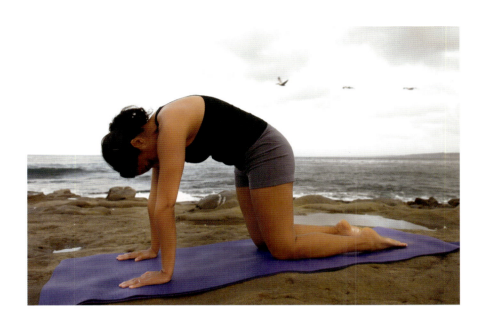

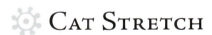 ## Cat Stretch

1. Begin on all fours with your belly pulled in and your limbs square. Drop your chin so that your neck is in line with your spine.
2. Exhale as you round your back like a cat while pulling your abs in. Inhale to drop the back into an arch while lifting the tail bone. Do not allow your belly to sag.

Purpose: To strengthen the back, increase mobility of the spine, and improve breathing

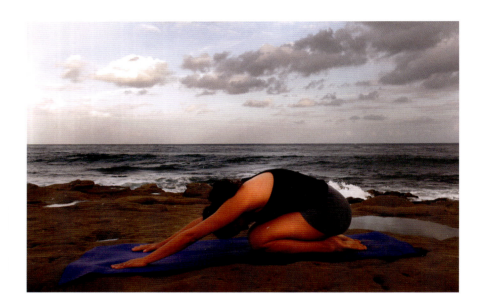

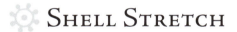 SHELL STRETCH

1. Exhale and sit back on your heels; stretch out your arms or fold them under your head.

Purpose: to release tension in the back

INTERMEDIATE/ADVANCED EXERCISE SEQUENCE

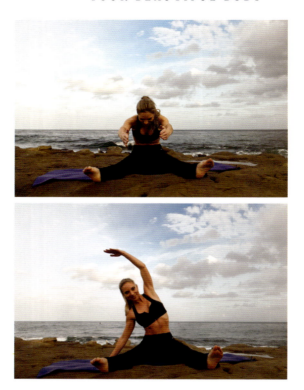

☼ Spine Stretch Forward plus Side Stretch

1. Sit up with the legs straight and open, shoulder width apart.
2. Inhale and pull the belly in. Exhale to roll forward as you reach the arms forward, as though sliding them along an imaginary shelf.
3. Inhale and roll back up, restacking the spine one vertebra at a time.
4. Then take one hand beside you, and stretch it up and over the head. Feel the stretch through your side.

Purpose: To stretch the back, hamstrings, and sides of torso
Reps: 4

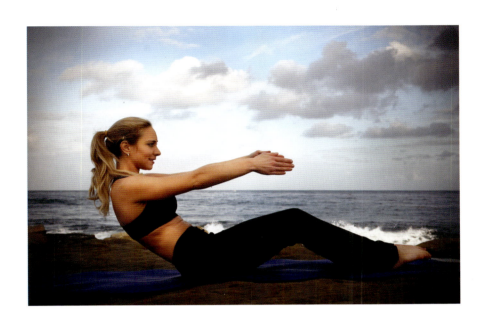

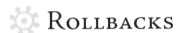 ## Rollbacks

1. Sit up with legs bent, arms in front of you.
2. Inhale, flatten the back and pull your abs in. Exhale, round your back like a c-curve and roll back, halfway down. Use your abs to keep you from falling.
3. Inhale, roll back up to the starting position.

Purpose: to strengthen the core and increase flexibility of the spine
Reps: 10

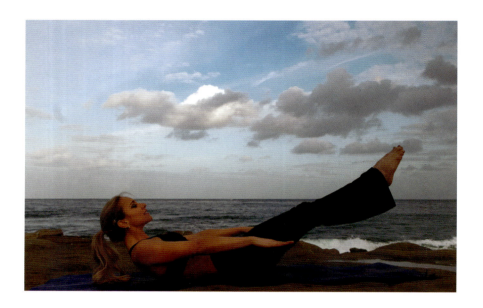

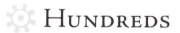 Hundreds

1. Lie on your back with the legs straight up and your arms above your head. Make sure your back is imprinted into the mat. Inhale.
2. Exhale; roll up the head, neck and shoulders, and pulse the arms by your sides.
3. Drop the legs lower to the floor to challenge the abs. If the lower back lifts off the mat, you know you have dropped the legs too far.
4. Inhale for 5 arm pulses, exhale for 5.

Purpose: to strengthen the abs
Reps: work up to 100 arm pulses

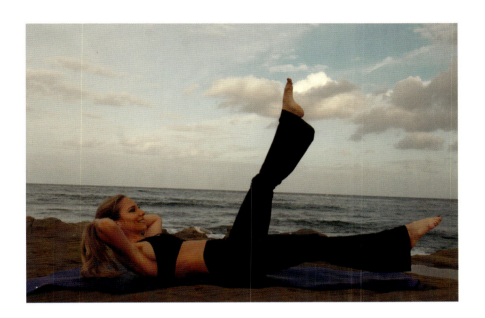

✹ Scissors Kicks

1. Lie on your back with your legs pointed straight up, arms beside you.
2. Keep your back on the mat and engage your abs.
3. Exhale as you kick the like scissors, slowly and with control. Feel your abs engage with each kick. Make the kicks only as large as you can keep your back on the mat and pelvis stable.

Purpose: to strengthen the abs, pelvic stability
Reps: 10-15 kicks

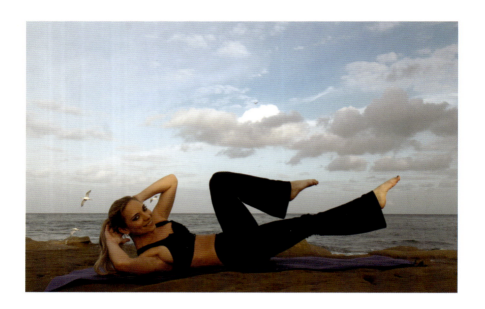

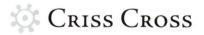 # Criss Cross

1. Lie on your back with your arms by your sides and your legs in a 90 degree angle.
2. Keep your back touching the mat and your abs engaged as you move the legs as though riding a bicycle. Crunch up, lifting the shoulder towards the opposite knee.
3. Exhale every time you crunch up. Feel the torso stabilize through the motion.

Purpose: to strengthen abs.
Reps: 10 times then repeat, working up to 20

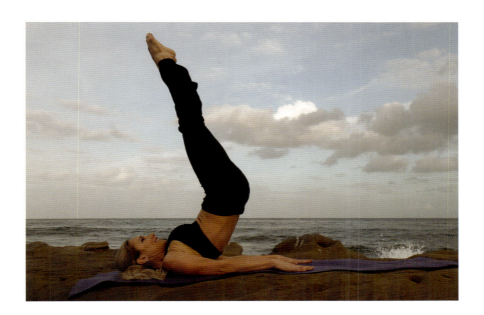

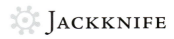 Jackknife

1. Lie on your back with your legs straight up, and your hands resting beside you.
2. Exhale as you roll your hips off the mat in a controlled way. It is ok for the arms to help you here, if needed.

Purpose: to strengthen the back and abs, and increase spinal flexion
Reps: 10

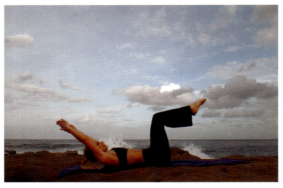

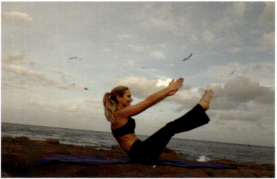

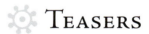 # Teasers

1. Lie on your back with your legs in a 90 degree angle, and your arms resting beside you.
2. Inhale; reach your arms above your head. Exhale; roll all the way up as the legs extend. Inhale; roll back down to starting.
3. Make sure your roll up smoothly, in control. Try to flatten the back at the top, then round the back to roll back down again. Pause slightly at the top.

Purpose: to strengthen the abs and back, hamstring flexibility
Reps: 8

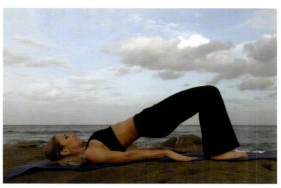
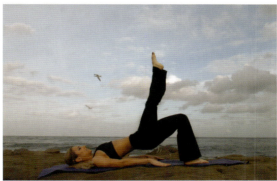

☼ Bridging and Single Leg Bridgings

1. Lie on your back with your knees bent, feet flat on the floor, arms beside you.
2. Exhale; roll the hips up towards the ceiling one vertebra at a time. Inhale to return.
3. Now extend one leg straight up, while keeping the hips level. Exhale; roll the hips up towards the ceiling by pushing off the single leg.

Purpose: to strengthen the legs, increase pelvic mobility
Reps: 8 both legs, then 8 more on each single leg

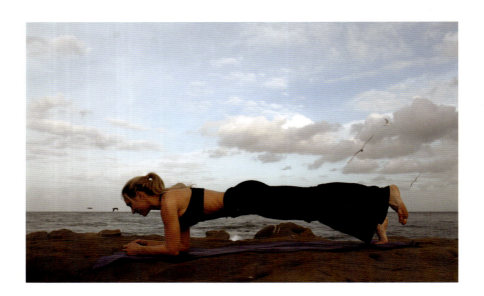

✦ Front Planks plus Side Leg

1. Begin face-down, on your toes and elbows. Keep your hips in line with your shoulders, so that the body is flat like a board.
2. Exhale; move one leg to the side, along the floor 8 times, then switch legs. Keep your body absolutely steady.

Purpose: core and shoulder strength
Reps: Hold for 30 seconds- 1 minute, then add legs

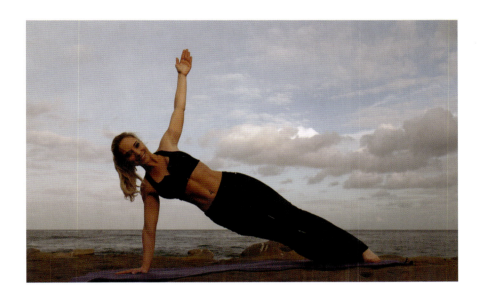

☼ Side Planks plus Hip Lift

1. Begin on your side with your elbow and lower knee (or feet) on the mat, top arm resting on your hip.
2. Exhale; lower hip towards floor. Inhale; lift hip towards ceiling. Continue the motion without resting on the floor.
3. Focus on feeling it deep in the lower side, and in the supporting shoulder.

Purpose: to strengthen abs, obliques, and shoulder. Get rid of muffin tops!
Reps: 10 each side

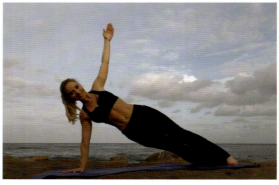

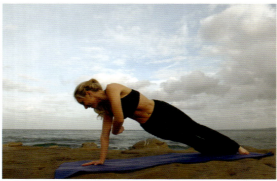

☼ Side Plank Twist (Snake)

1. Begin on the side, supported by one hand and your feet. Reach the top arm towards the ceiling.
2. Exhale; reach the top hand underneath your armpit while twisting the from the torso. Return.
3. Keep your lower body steady and look where you are going as you twist.

Purpose: to strengthen the abs and obliques. Get rid of muffin tops!

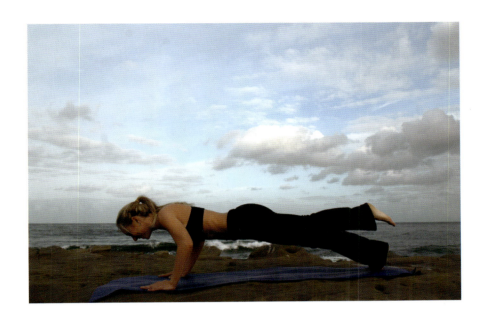

☼ Extra Fun Push Ups

1. Begin in push-up position with one leg lifted behind you. Keep that leg lifted as you work through the set, hips level.

Purpose: to strengthen the upper body and core
Reps: 8-15

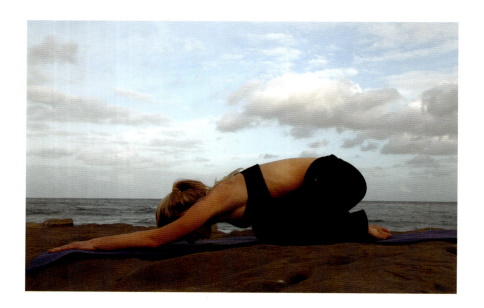

☼ Shell Stretch

1. Begin in all fours position.
2. Sit back on your heels with arms stretched out in front of you. Relax any tension out of your back. Breathe normally.

Purpose: to stretch the back
Hold 20 seconds

CHAPTER FOUR

PILATES FOR REHABILITATION AND PREVENTION OF BACK PAIN

"Every human being is the author of his own health or disease."

    ❦ BUDDHA

Low-back pain is the most common cause of job-related disability in the United States, according to the National Institute of Neurological Disorders and Stroke. Approximately 80% of people will experience back pain at some point in their lives. Chronic back pain causes people to miss work and affects their daily activities. Keeping your body healthy with Pilates can prevent back pain and help you feel stronger year after year.

WHAT CAUSES BACK PAIN?

Back pain can be caused by a variety of conditions; however, the most common cause is poor posture. How you hold your body during movement, sitting at your desk, and even sleeping can create muscular imbalances in your body. Often repetitive stress from sitting at a desk all day, poor posture, or an unsupportive mattress will be the initial cause of your back pain.

Spending all day sitting at a desk in front of a computer is a common source of back problems. Unfortunately, most people work under these conditions and they find it very difficult to sit up with proper posture for eight hours at a time. It becomes a vicious cycle. First you sit for long periods of time in a way that doesn't properly support the spine (generally, in a slightly hunched-over position). Then you lose strength in your postural muscles by not using them day after day, and then you can't sit up properly even if you wanted to because you've lost strength! On top of that, poor posture tends to make some muscles tighter, and the opposing muscles weaker, causing an imbalance in the body. What to do? Well, guess what? Pilates!

A sedentary lifestyle may also be to blame. It is difficult to use good posture for any length of time, and the body starts to hunch forward. (I am reminding myself to sit up straighter as I write this). If you think about it, when you sit in a chair, the back muscles have to work all the time to keep you upright. Your legs are not able to help out at all. Furthermore, staying in one position doesn't promote good circulation and muscle tone.

Break up your work day by getting up regularly from your chair and stretching out, going for a walk, or doing a Pilates series, if you can. I often tell my clients to set a timer to remind them to get up and move around every hour. If you can practice sitting in good posture, and strengthen the muscles that support the spine, then you will be able to sit in a healthy posture. Hunching forward just won't feel right anymore!

Be aware that there are several more serious causes of back pain, such as sprain or strain of tendons and ligaments, herniated discs, or other degenerative diseases of the spine. As we age, the inter-vertebral discs of the spine degenerate and become less lubricated, losing their ability to support the back well. Sitting in a chair for long periods at a time and a lack of physical activity accelerates this process. These discs begin to compress the nerves that exit between each vertebrae causing pain, tingling, or numbness.

Back pain can be very frustrating and take a toll on everyday activities. The best action is to prevent pain and injury before it starts by sitting with a good posture, doing core exercises, and moving around throughout the day.

PILATES HELPS TO CORRECT POSTURE

Joseph Pilates' system was originally called Contrology and was primarily developed to help rehabilitate injuries and strengthen the body. Pilates focuses on strengthening the core muscles of the body, which includes the abdomen, hips, and lower back. These muscle groups support our posture and prevent injury, especially to the lower back.

It is more likely to injure the spine if it has lost strength and flexibility. Since Pilates focuses on the development of strength and flexibility in a controlled manner, it can rehabilitate and prevent back injury. Pilates exercises, such as the ones in this book, will strengthen your core muscles and correct muscles imbalances in your body.

In Pilates, we pay a lot of attention to how our body parts are lined up in relation to each other; our alignment. When alignment is off, uneven stress is on the skeleton, especially the spine. This causes muscular imbalances, and ultimately pain. Pilates exercises, done with attention to alignment, create uniform muscle use and development, and allow the body to work in a natural and healthy way.

The Pilates method will help to engage the core muscles. This is accomplished by pulling the navel towards the spine, and slightly tucking under the hips. As you adjust your body in this manner, the core muscles begin to support your torso and align the posture. This technique should be used while you exercise, walk, sit or stand. Examples of this are in the exercise section.

Correct your posture by following these guidelines:

- Do not stand or walk with your knees locked, which can create unnecessary pressure on your spine.

- Make sure to engage your abdominal muscles at all times, keeping your core strong will help the deep stabilizing muscles of the body support your weight.

- Keep your shoulders pulled down and back while standing tall. Maintaining this vertical alignment will decrease stress in the neck and shoulder area, and will allow the muscles to work efficiently.

- Learn to keep your pelvis in a neutral position. One of the most common postural imbalances that people have is the tendency to either tuck or tilt the pelvis. Both positions create weaknesses on one side of the body and overly tighten areas on the other. These imbalances lead to misalignment, and cause pain with time and use. Doing Pilates with correct pelvic alignment can strengthen the muscles in a balanced way, decreasing pain, especially in the back.

Check Your Own Posture!

Stand naturally so that you have a side view of your body in a mirror. You should be able to make an imaginary line that connects the tip of your ear to your shoulder, the top of your pelvis, the side of the knee, down to the front of your ankle bone. Figure A. If your belly pooches out and your back arches, then you know that you need to strengthen your abdominals, for example. Figure B. If your shoulders and head are rounded forward, then you know you need to strengthen your back, as shown in Figure C. A sway back, as illustrated in Figure D, represents a person with scoliosis. A better view of this can be seen in Figure E.

Each of these spinal deviations can be improved with the correct exercise programs. Fortunately, the Pilates exercises described in this book can help all of these deviations when done with precision and good form. Be aware of your posture throughout the day!

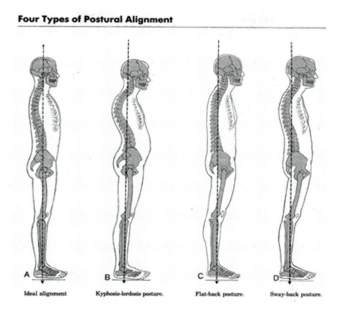

Four Types of Postural Alignment

A. Ideal alignment. B. Kyphosis-lordosis posture. C. Flat-back posture. D. Sway-back posture.

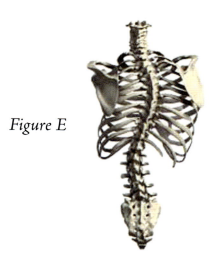

Figure E

The main things to remember to prevent bad posture are to sit and stand up tall, keep your belly pulled in, and keep your shoulder blades pulling down your back. Practicing good posture will become natural over time, and will prevent pain and imbalance in the body.

PILATES DEVELOPS CORE STRENGTH

Having great core strength helps to relieve and prevent back pain. Core strength means that all of the muscles of the trunk of your body are strong, flexible, and working together to support and stabilize the spine.

Muscles of the core go much deeper than the famous "6 pack" muscles. The abdominals, back and deep muscles of the pelvis all play a role in core strength. Traditional forms of exercise tend to focus on the larger, more superficial muscle groups. And while this is important, it does not have the same affect that Pilates does on strengthening the deep layers of muscle that support the spine, and play a role in every movement. Complete core strength and mobility are essential for back health.

Some of the important core muscles are the ones located on the pelvic floor; the psoas, which play a huge role in keeping us upright and in hip bending; the spinalis, which are small muscles that weave along the spine; and the transverse and oblique abdominal muscles. The diaphragm, our prime breathing muscle, is right in the middle of the core. All of these muscles play crucial roles in the support and stability of the spine.

"...the only real guide to your true age lies not in years or how you THINK you feel but as you ACTUALLY are as infallibly indicated by the natural and normal flexibility enjoyed by your spine..." - Joseph Pilates

The important principles of Pilates are consistent with an exercise program that promotes back health. In particular, learning awareness of neutral alignment of the spine and strengthening the deep postural muscles that support this alignment are important skills for the back pain patient.

Patients with pain stemming from degeneration of the discs and joints are particularly likely to benefit from a Pilates exercise program. In addition, as the posture improves, the balance of the muscles improves, thus decreasing wear and tear resulting from uneven stresses on the joints and discs.

Pilates improves strength, flexibility and suppleness of the muscles of the hip and shoulder girdle. As the strength and mobility of the joints improves, there is more fluid to help the joints move without pain, and more muscle to support the joint in a healthy position.

The Pilates program teaches body awareness. It can improve how you use your body, how you sit, and how you breathe. This awareness decreases tension and helps you to use the body efficiently.

PILATES PROMOTES FLEXIBILITY

A healthy spine can curve forward and backward, twist, and move side to side. Strengthening the core muscles forms a protective support for the spine, and increases its range of motion. Pilates' exercises are easy to modify so that we can develop spinal flexibility at our own pace. This is one of the things about Pilates that makes it easy for people with back pain to work with.

CONSIDERATIONS FOR
BACK PAIN PATIENTS

Before starting any new exercise system, it is always advisable to check with a physician or other healthcare provider. Most doctors and physical therapists now recommend Pilates for patients needing rehabilitation with a certified professional.

Individuals with significant back problems may benefit from several one-on-one Pilates sessions with a qualified Pilates instructor. Private sessions can be more costly than classes, but are well worth the investment. Learning to do the exercises correctly will ensure that you are helping the problem rather than making it worse. Eventually you may find that you will be able to enter a class with the security in knowing that you are performing the exercises correctly. Some clients may benefit from twice per week sessions, and then decrease that to once a week to maintain results.

PILATES HAS A WAY OF MAKING THE SIMPLEST EXERCISES EFFECTIVE

You cannot underestimate the benefit of simple exercises that support the deep postural muscles of the trunk, awareness of neutral alignment, and healthy mobility of the shoulders and hips.

Pilates originates as a method of rehabilitation, but also has roots in ballet and dance. A lot of the exercises are difficult and may be inappropriate for clients with back pain or degenerative disc disease. As a general rule, back patients should avoid exercises that push the spine into extremes of flexion or extension, or combine flexion with side bending or twisting the spine. These motions place excessive stress on the discs.

The exercises in the Pilates system should be both mentally and physically challenging but not so difficult that they cause you to struggle. If the exercise causes pain, then it may be too difficult, or the person may need additional help to do it correctly.

AVOIDING LOADED FLEXION

Most women who have office jobs have back problems by the time they're in their 40's because they spend much of their day sitting hunched over a desk. They spend countless hours with their head forward, and their backs rounded with little support for their vertebrae. Likewise, professional movers develop back issues after bending over lifting heavy objects over and over. Even if you maintain perfect alignment when lifting, you can't avoid loading the spine in flexion if you're lifting heavy objects (like a toddler!) or doing much of anything below the waist.

Flexion is the rounding forward of the spine when standing or sitting, or what your spine does when rolling up in a sit up. *Loaded* means lifting any sort of weight. An example of loading the spine in flexion is standing with a heavy book in your hands and then leaning over with it. The muscles and ligaments of the back are supporting that weight. When you get very strong in your core, your spine can support more weight without being traumatized. Flexion is the movement of the spine that most damages the structures of the spine, and therefore it is important to strengthen your back to prevent injury. If you feel uncomfortable when doing flexion exercises; don't do them! Instead, do all the exercises that don't bother your back, and come back to the others when you have more strength. When in doubt, stick with the exercises that feel right and avoid the ones that cause pain or discomfort.

Remember, if you have to lift something heavy, engage your abs to support your back and let your legs do the work. Don't round the back; keep it straight. Lifting and bending with proper form can prevent a back injury that can sometimes happen with minimal effort.

Listen to your body as you proceed with Pilates, or any other form of exercise. It takes time to see the benefit of the work, but with time it will become apparent. You will probably gain strength and mobility early, and it won't take long for your exercise routine to make a positive difference in your life, and in your mood.

TIPS FOR DECREASING BACK PAIN

Breathing

Practice deep breathing during an acute attack of back pain. This will help to calm your mind, send oxygen to the muscles, and will allow the body to relax.

Lie on a Hard Surface

Lying on the floor with your knees bent and propped up by a pillow can decrease pressure on your lower back. The hard surface supports the spine in a way that helps to relieve pain and pressure on the spine.

Stretch Often

Remember to get up and move at least every hour. Do light stretching several times per day to prevent your body from becoming stiff. Stretching and moving will also increase the circulation and will help to send more blood and nutrients to your back.

Don't Sit for Long Periods of Time

Sitting for long periods of time is a common cause of back pain. A poor sitting posture is typical during long work hours, which leads to repetitive stress on the muscles causing muscle imbalances. Pull your abs in, sit tall, and breathe. Good posture will help to prevent muscle strain. I have even recommended using a timer at your desk to remind you to get up and move every hour. It works!

Pilates Increases Body Awareness

Look on the bright side. Having back pain makes us more aware of our bodies and how we move. Whether the cause of pain is from an injury or a culmination of the effects of poor posture and inefficient movement habits, back pain is a messenger letting us know that we need to pay more attention to the way we live. Doing Pilates makes us more aware of our alignment and how we move. This is a valuable tool to have as we go on about our busy lives, and continue to age…. gracefully of course.

KEY ELEMENTS TO MAKING YOUR WORKOUT EFFECTIVE

Strengthening the abdominals and the muscles that support the spine will go a long way in decreasing and preventing back pain. Often, back pain is caused or aggravated by weak abdominals which push out away from the spine, leaving little support for your back. It is very important to combat this by learning to pull your abdominals in while gently tucking your buttocks underneath you. This helps to lengthen the back and tighten the abdominals. The goal is to "imprint" your back onto the mat when you are lying down. This is the safest, most effective position to workout. At the same time, lengthen your neck by gently dropping your chin, and dropping your shoulders. This will relieve stress and tightness in your neck and upper back. Keep the focus in your core, and relax the tightness out of your upper body.

Start with the Beginning exercise section which is demonstrated by Laura Otero. Do the exercises in order. No exercise should cause pain. If you ever find that an exercise is putting uncomfortable strain or pain in your body, then stop. Make sure you are doing the exercise correctly. If it still causes pain, then skip the exercise for now and move on to something that feels right. Listen to your body as you perform the work. Remember, doing the exercises should relieve pain, give you energy, and make you feel good!

CHAPTER FIVE

ANTI-AGING STRATEGIES FOR A LEAN AND BEAUTIFUL BODY

"Excellence is not a singular act, but a habit. You are what you repeatedly do."
❖ SHAQUILLE O'NEAL

Let's address some key factors to help you look and feel young, even as you age. As we get older, our bodies change. We start to lose bone and muscle and our metabolism slows, causing weight gain. Our skin becomes duller, and our immune system starts to weaken. It is possible to prevent a lot of this if you take a few simple steps in the right direction that will help you maintain your youth!

1. YOUR METABOLISM

Metabolism is the rate at which your body burns calories. There are a few factors that influence your metabolism, including your basal metabolic rate, how much muscle mass you have, and how much and when you eat. Each of these plays a key role in determining whether you will maintain, lose, or gain weight with age. Did you know that your metabolism slows by about 5% each decade after the age of 25? That means that if you are 45, then you burn about 200 calories fewer each day than you did when you were in your twenties. Not good for the waistline, or your mood, but don't fret! We are not destined to this fate!

During the complex biochemical process of metabolism, calories in food and beverage are combined with oxygen to release the energy your body needs to function. The body needs energy when you are at rest to breath, circulate blood, adjust hormone levels, and to grow and repair cells. The number of calories your body uses to carry out these basic functions is known as your basal metabolic rate (BMR). We will talk about this in a later chapter, including how to calculate how many calories you should be eating to lose weight. Your BMR accounts for 60-75% of how many calories you burn each day.

BMR is determined by factors such as:

❧ Your Body Size- larger people burn more calories, even at rest.

❧ Your Sex- men usually burn more calories than women because they have more muscle mass.

❧ Your Age- As you age, you tend to lose muscle and gain fat, slowing down your body's ability to burn calories.

It is tempting to blame your metabolism for weight gain. However, our metabolism naturally balances to the needs of our body. That is why your metabolism slows down if you try a starvation diet. Your body will compensate for the lack of calories by slowing down to conserve those calories for survival. Unfortunately, weight gain is most commonly the result of eating more calories than you burn. To lose weight, you must eat fewer calories and also burn more calories by doing physical activity.

Fire up Your Metabolism with Physical Activity

Your metabolism starts to slow down as you become less active and your body starts to lose muscle. You can combat the loss of muscle and consequently this decrease in your metabolic rate by increasing your physical activity. Everything counts such as playing tennis, walking the dog, or chasing the kids. All of these activities will help you burn more calories each day. You can control the number of calories you burn in a day; the

ANTI-AGING STRATEGIES FOR A LEAN AND BEAUTIFUL BODY 69

more active you are the more calories you burn. In fact, fidgety people who appear to have a higher metabolism are actually just more active!

You can burn more calories by:

Regular Aerobic Exercise. Go for a walk or get on that exercise equipment! Keep it going for at least 30-40 minutes a day to boost your calorie burn. Even if you can't find the time, do three or four bursts of 10-minute activity. It will have the same effect!

Strength Training or Pilates. This is extremely important to combat the decrease in metabolism associated with muscle loss. Muscle tissue burns more calories than fat tissue does, so it's imperative to strengthen your muscles as you age. Keep your muscles toned by lifting weights, or doing Pilates, and it will help to keep your metabolism revved!

Lifestyle Activities. Any extra movement will burn calories, so get off the couch and do something already! Become a professional at keeping your house clean! Do squats or pushups off the counter while you cook dinner!

Fire up Your Metabolism through Eating

Don't Skip Breakfast! Or Any Meal for that Matter. It always amazes me how people who want to lose weight try to do so by skipping meals, especially breakfast. Then they wonder why their diets never work. That's because skipping meals is a big mistake. When your body is deprived of food, it starts conserving fuel by burning fewer calories. Then when you do eat, your body will store more as fat in preparation for the next famine. Skipping breakfast sets your body into this famine mode, and makes it difficult to lose weight, or keep your body fat low. Since your metabolism slows down while you are sleeping, the first thing you should do is give it a jump-start by eating something small in the morning. A banana and half a cup of orange juice is a great choice or a nonfat yogurt and piece of whole wheat toast.

Eat Throughout the Day. The types of people who skip breakfast and skimp on calories in the first half of the day also tend to eat a large meal at night. These types of eaters usually have more body fat, especially in their middle. The body is not made to process fuel efficiently when you overeat at one meal. Eating small portions throughout the day allows the body's metabolism to work efficiently, the blood sugar to remain stable, and keeps the body primed for movement. Did I mention that these types of "grazers" have less body fat? The trick is to spread your meals out during your day. If you pack a turkey sandwich, an apple, and some cookies for your lunch then eat the apple at 11:00, the sandwich at noon, and the cookies at 1:00. By the time you are thinking about dinner you won't be so starving that you will binge on the first thing in sight.

Being Aware of Portion Size. Research shows that eating large portions in one meal overloads your system which messes up your digestion and packs on unwanted body fat. Instead, eat less at every sitting, and plan on eating more often throughout your day. It isn't easy when America's restaurants super size everything, and make it extra tempting with a good price. After all, for only 20 cents more, you can get the 24-ounce soda rather than the 16-ounce soda. It is a better deal, but not for your waistline. A typical serving of pasta in a restaurant has enough servings to feed four people, not one. Defend yourself against the overeating epidemic by having your server put half of your order in a to-go box *before* they bring it out. It is much less tempting, and will be perfect for lunch the next day. Also, have a cup of broth-based soup or small side salad before your entrée. You will be less likely to overeat when your meal arrives.

Close the Kitchen by 8:00 p.m. It is a myth that a meal eaten late at night will make you gain weight. In fact, it doesn't matter if you eat that pasta at 5 p.m. or at 8 p.m.; your body does not metabolize food more slowly at night than it does in the day. Weight gain happens when you consume more calories than you burn, regardless of when you eat them. However, late-night nibblers tend to consume more calories which can add up to unwanted pounds. Mindless eating in front of the TV can cause you to consume more calories than you thought. The people who don't eat enough during the day tend to overeat at night. Eat a lot of mini meals throughout the day to prevent binge-eating at night. Also try to eat dinner before 6 p.m. so that your body has time to digest it before you go to bed. That way you will wake up hungry and ready to jump-start your body with a light breakfast! I also try to limit my carbohydrate intake after 6 p.m. Eating foods such as lean protein and veggies or fruit in the evening will let you wake up without feeling bloated.

2. EAT YOUR WAY TO BEAUTIFUL SKIN

Healthy eating leads to healthy skin. Of course it is extremely important that we stay out of the sun and use good skin care, but what we consume plays a major role on how our skin will look and feel as we age. Loading up on plenty of fruits and vegetables will give your body the nutrients it needs to have young, supple skin, and combat free radicals. Free radicals are harmful substances found in pollution, cigarette smoke, herbicides, radiation, fried foods and other unhealthy things. Basically, they are molecules with unpaired electrons. These molecules attack our healthy cells looking for an electron to steal, thereby causing our cells to become damaged and defenseless. This can lead to many diseases, including cancer. Normally, the body can neutralize free radicals as long as it has antioxidants available. Since free radical damage accumulates with age, it is extremely important that we get plenty of antioxidants into our diet now. The following nutrients are part of a balanced, healthy-skin diet:

Vitamins C and E protect the body against the destructive effects of free radicals which to contributes to aging skin. Antioxidant-rich foods that are high in vitamin C include red bell peppers, oranges, broccoli, mango and strawberries. Foods high in vitamin E include peanuts, almonds, sunflower seeds and hazelnuts.

Vitamin B (biotin) helps to form the foundation of our hair, skin, and nails. It is in turkey, oats, Brazil nuts, potatoes, avocados, bananas and legumes.

Vitamin A helps to maintain and repair skin tissue, eyesight, and minimizes wrinkles and sun spots. Eat carrots, yams (my favorite!), spinach, cantaloupe, dark green and yellow vegetables, milk, eggs and cheese.

Lean protein, especially proteins that contain Omega-3's, decrease inflammation and plays a role in your skin's structure and function. Fuel up on wild salmon, healthy oils, and nuts.

Drinking enough **water** is crucially important to maintain supple skin. Lack of hydration leads to dry, flaky skin that looks more wrinkled. Just imagine a raisin! Aim to drink at least 8 glasses of water a day for your skin.

Eating more fruits and veggies is one of the best things you can do for your body! Not only will your skin thank you, so will your waistline. Ideally, we should eat 5-8 servings of fruits and veggies every day. Keep them available in your fridge or freezer and include them at every meal. It is easy and delicious! Check out some of the recipes at the end of the book for great ideas to increasing your vegetable intake.

3. TAKE SUPPLEMENTS AS AN INSURANCE POLICY FOR YOUR HEALTH

It is ideal to get your nutrients from eating a healthy balanced diet that provides most of the vitamins and minerals that your body needs. These nutrients can be absorbed and utilized more completely when they come from whole food sources, rather than a supplement. However, it is not always possible to eat perfectly all the time, so taking a multivitamin is a great way to cover all of your bases when it comes to getting in your daily allowance of vitamins and minerals. Think about it as an insurance policy for your health. A good multivitamin will provide at least 100

ANTI-AGING STRATEGIES FOR A LEAN AND BEAUTIFUL BODY   73

percent of the recommended daily allowance (RDA) for most nutrients and trace minerals. Your body doesn't need more than the RDA, and taking more than that for fat-soluble nutrients like vitamins A, D and K could cause harm.

Vitamins C and E are important for their immune and antioxidant properties as I mentioned earlier, so make sure they are included in your multivitamin. The RDA for Vitamin E is 30IU, and 60mg for Vitamin C. Taking extra of these nutrients should only help you, but be sure to consult your doctor for his or her recommendation.

In addition to taking a daily multivitamin, it is important to add a calcium supplement, especially for women. Most multivitamins don't have nearly enough calcium, so taking an extra supplement is important. It is recommended to pick a calcium supplement that supplies at least 500 mg, as it is optimal for most women to take 1,000 mg per day. Vitamin D and Vitamin K are also thought to play a role in the absorption of calcium, and some calcium supplements include them. Milk, salmon and tuna are excellent sources of Vitamin D. My favorite calcium supplement is Viactiv; the caramel chews taste like candy! Taking calcium helps your bones stay strong as you age. Studies have shown that women who consume at least 750 mg of calcium daily reduce their chances of getting a hip fracture by 60 percent. Not getting enough calcium leads to osteoporosis which causes your bones to become thin, brittle, and weak. Half of American women over the age of 65 have osteoporosis, so start taking your supplement now to prevent excessive bone loss! Normally, women reach their peak bone density at the end of their 20's. After that, most of us start to lose bone density at a slow rate. That rate escalates as women hit menopause and their estrogen production stops. Factors other than calcium intake affect the rate of bone loss such as exercise, eating habits, smoking and drinking. Women who do regular weight-baring exercises such as walking, playing tennis, or even gardening have stronger bones than those who don't. So take your calcium and get out for a walk, and you will save your bones as you age!

4. EAT FOODS RICH WITH FIBER

Fiber is a substance that is found in plants that does not breakdown during the digestive process Most people have heard about how good it is to get enough fiber in your diet, but they do not all understand how or why it is so important. We should all be eating about 25-30 grams of fiber a day, but most of us consume only half of that.

There are two kinds of fiber:

- Insoluble fiber cannot be dissolved in water. It aids in digestion by speeding up the passage of foods through your stomach and intestines. It relieves constipation and hemorrhoids.

- Soluble fiber can be absorbed by water. It stabilizes blood sugar levels by slowing down the digestion of carbohydrates, and reduces cholesterol levels.

A diet rich in fiber can lower your risk of developing:

Heart disease and high cholesterol. Soluble fiber helps to lower cholesterol levels in the blood which helps to minimize the risk for getting heart disease. Heart disease is the leading cause of death for both men and women, according to the Centers for Disease Control (CDC). That is a good enough reason to increase your fiber intake!

Cancer. Fiber speeds up the passage of food through the body and therefore eliminates the absorption of unhealthy substances found in some foods that may play a role in colon cancer. Other types of cancer including breast cancer, ovarian cancer and uterine cancer may also benefit from a diet rich in fiber.

Diabetes. Fiber helps to regulate blood sugar levels which are important in avoiding diabetes. It also helps to reduce blood sugar, and can help people with diabetes reduce their medication.

Constipation and Hemorrhoids. Fiber helps to relieve constipation within hours by softening the stool. It aids in the health of the colon and helps to prevent Hemorrhoids.

Periodontal Disease. Fibrous foods that are crunchy such as nuts, raw carrots and apples can help your teeth and gums stay healthy so that you are less likely to develop this disease.

Fiber also helps you lose and maintain a healthy weight! It makes you feel full so that you eat less overall. It acts as a natural appetite suppressant! A diet high in fiber is important in staying lean by reducing your overall calorie intake, and helping digestion. Fill up on whole fiber-filled foods in their natural form. For example, instead of taking a supplement, choose foods that contain fiber. Avoid foods that have had the fiber removed, such as fruit juice. It is high in calories and sugar, and completely void of fiber. It is much better for your waistline and your health to eat that apple or orange in its fresh and whole form.

Here are some foods to help you increase your fiber intake while helping you lose weight:

Insoluble fiber can be found in:

- Green beans

- Dark, leafy vegetables

- Asparagus

- Cauliflower

- Zucchini

- Beets

- Celery

- Whole grain breads
- Whole wheat
- Wheat bran
- Fruit skins
- Pears
- Seeds
- Nuts

Soluble fiber can be found in:

- Carrots
- Broccoli
- Dried beans
- Peas
- Oat bran
- Barley
- Rye
- Flaxseed
- Nuts
- Oranges
- Apples
- Prunes
- Plums

ANTI-AGING STRATEGIES FOR A LEAN AND BEAUTIFUL BODY   77

Fiber has so many benefits, so start today by adding some of these foods to your diet and watch your health improve and your weight go down.

5. WATER IS YOUR FOUNTAIN OF YOUTH

Water is truly a magical substance. It aids in countless processes of bodily function, and helps us to lose weight. It aids in the digestion process, and like fiber, it keeps us feeling full longer. In fact, you can't lose weight or keep your skin beautiful or your body healthy without it! Did you know that you are already dehydrated by the time you feel thirsty? The body needs at least 10 glasses of water daily to maintain its function. If you exercise or drink caffeinated beverages, then you need even more. Try to aim for an extra glass of water for every cup of coffee or caffeinated beverage you consume. Without water, your heart has to work harder to pump blood to your brain and heart, and your skin will look wrinkled like a raisin.

Try these tricks to stay hydrated and keep your body functioning well. Drink a tall glass of water in the morning when you get up, and again before every meal. It will help you get enough water throughout the day, and will curb your appetite before you eat! It's easy to forget to drink water throughout the day because we can get caught up in our daily activities. That is why taking a bottle of water everywhere you go can be helpful. If you see it sitting on your desk beside you, or next to you in the car, you will remember to drink it. Another idea is to set a timer every 30 minutes or hour to remind you to drink a glass of water. Don't worry if you have to go to the bathroom more often; that's your chance to take a walk. Besides, it's worth that small hassle to feel more energized, enjoy youthful skin, and have your weight loss goals achieved. So drink up!

What if you can't stand the taste of water? Ok, first you will like it more if you practice drinking it. However, there are other options that may help you. Try drinking seltzer with a splash or cranberry juice, ice water with lemon slices, unsweetened green tea, or Crystal Light. These beverages offer the hydration of water with extra flavor, and little or no calories.

6. LIMIT YOUR CONSUMPTION OF SWEETS AND SALTY SNACKS

I love sugar and anything that has to do with chocolate or ice cream. It is hard for me to resist eating sweets, and I rarely get through the day without them. I know you have your favorites too; some of my clients admit to loving sweets, while others admit to craving salty foods. Whatever your craving is, I want you to know that you do not have to give it up to look fabulous and still be healthy and fit. You just have to eat them in moderation. I know you have heard this before, but let's talk about what that really means.

Nutrition experts tell us that less than 10% of our daily caloric intake should be from sugary foods. That means that you should not consume more than 160 calories from sweets if you are on a 1600 calorie diet. That isn't much! Take a look at a small candy bar from the grocery store checkout line; most have more than 200 calories. A small bag of Doritos will also cost you about 200 calories, and you will only get about 15 chips. It is worth watching the amount of calories we consume in the form of sweets and salty snacks, because they add up fast! Why not eat a nonfat yogurt with some frozen berries and a sprinkle of chocolate chips? You will be far more satisfied, and will get valuable nutrition too.

Here is more must-read advice to deal with cravings:

- Practice choosing nutritional sweet foods over processed sugary or salty foods. Bite into a crunchy apple or luscious peach instead of that bowl of ice cream. I know it's not nearly as tempting, but you will be glad you made that choice as soon as your teeth sink into it, and even more glad when you wake up the next morning.

ANTI-AGING STRATEGIES FOR A LEAN AND BEAUTIFUL BODY 79

❧ It is usually easier to start your day off on the right track rather than end it that way. I make sure to eat a light healthy breakfast and lunch from my foods list that we will talk about in Chapter 7. That way I don't have to feel guilty about indulging in a serving of ice cream or a bar of chocolate later in the day when I want it the most. Indulging in this way every day also prevents me from bingeing on sweets later. You see, I have tried to avoid this afternoon sweet attack many times, and have also failed many times. It only makes me feel guilty and defeated, and the results are always the same. I now look forward to my small treat every day, knowing that it is part of my daily caloric budget. I can maintain my healthy weight and still enjoy life… in moderation.

❧ Sweets are very addictive. The more you eat, the more you want. Researchers have found that the taste of refined sugar creates a craving for more refined sugar. Since sugary foods are usually low in fiber and nutrition, filling up on them is not a good idea. When a sugar or salt craving hits you, you may just be thirsty. Drink a tall glass of water and then see how you feel.

❧ Distraction is the key! Most of the time you start thinking about a craving because you are bored or listless. Use this time to do something you have been meaning to do. If your hands and brain are busy typing an email or scrubbing the toilet, you will be less likely to get into the snacks. It is amazing how you can forget about the cookies when you are running around doing other things!

❧ Don't leave home without a healthy snack. The only thing worse than trying to avoid a craving is when you're hungry on top of it. You know how it goes; it's the afternoon energy-crash and you are already feeling hungry. If you don't have a healthy snack on hand, then it makes it even more difficult to avoid the vending machine. Keep a bag of dried fruit, an apple, a low-sugar energy bar, or a container of fruit in your car or at your desk so that you are prepared when these times arise.

- A lot of companies are now offering your favorite treats in small 100-calorie packages. They are mini versions of the same product, and are individually packaged to help us avoid over-consumption. Keep some of these single serving packages around, and remember to eat only one!

- If you like chocolate, then splurge on purchasing expensive quality chocolate from your local confectioner, or chocolate like Godiva. You will feel like you are getting a treat as you enjoy a rich truffle or chocolate covered strawberry, and you will be more likely to be satisfied with just one.

- So what happens if you end up bingeing on that hot fudge sundae or eating an entire bag of chips? First, don't beat yourself up. We have all done it before. Just compensate by eating well the next day (or next week if it's holiday or vacation time) and put in a little extra time at the gym. You will not gain weight if you are generally eating healthy. Make good choices most of the time, and then you can enjoy your favorite sinful foods too.

7. CONSUME ALCOHOL IN MODERATION

Research has indicated that drinking one serving of alcohol for women (2 servings for men) per day may help prevent heart disease. A single serving of alcohol is a 5-ounce glass of wine, a 12-ounce beer, or 1.5 ounces of hard liquor. Drinking any more than this will only increase your risk for breast cancer, liver damage, cause you to be dehydrated, and gain weight. It's not worth over-indulging in alcohol.

Alcohol contains a significant amount of calories, and can cause you to gain weight if you over-indulge. You don't need to stop cold-turkey, but you do need to limit yourself to no more than one serving per day. In addition to being high in calories, alcohol softens our resolve to make healthy food choices, setting us up to eat more calories than we would have otherwise.

Alcohol acts as a diuretic, flushing water and nutrients out of your system much like coffee, soda, and other caffeinated beverages. Dehydration from drinking also leads to sagging, wrinkled skin and disrupted sleep patterns. You can counteract the effects of dehydration from alcohol and caffeinated beverages by drinking extra water. Drink an additional glass of water for every serving of alcohol consumed. In addition, drink a tall glass or bottle of water before you go to bed so that you can wake up fresh without a hangover or dull skin.

Personally, I would rather save drinking alcohol for parties or weekends, but some people love wine like I love sweets. If this is you, then I recommend limiting your intake to one serving per day, and flush it out with plenty of water.

CHAPTER SIX

D.I.E.T.:
DIVINE INSPIRATION FOR EVERYDAY TRIUMPHS

"I've been on a constant diet for the last two decades. I've lost a total of 789 pounds. By all accounts, I should be hanging from a charm bracelet."
❖ ERMA BOMBECK

When you think of the word Diet, what feelings come to mind? What thoughts do you have? What expressions would you use? I asked a few friends to play a little game with me and try to come up with a definition of the word Diet as if it was an acronym. What would D.I.E.T. stand for? Here were some of their responses.

Did I Eat That?

Doubt I Even Tried

Deprived of It Every Time

Do It Eventually Tomorrow

Daunting Insufferable Excuses Today

Decrease Indulgent Eating Temptations

After hearing all of these negative associations to the word, I challenged them to come up with positive terms that could change their mood and their outlook. What I was looking for were possible affirmations around the process of changing eating habits to support a healthy lifestyle. As you probably guessed, they groaned at the thought of even considering that there was a positive spin on this subject. I did not back down and here were a few of the final winners.

Divine Inspiration for Everyday Triumphs

Develop Interesting Exciting Tastes

Deeply Individual Emotional Triumph

Discovering Inspiration Eliminates Tension

Decisive Installment Efforts Treasured

Daily Intake of Exercise Triumphs

Can you think of any more acronyms? Email me at:

lariesa@pilatesofeastlake.com.

When I ask my clients what their diets consisted of I would usually hear an answer given with a proper name, such as South Beach, Zone, Atkins, Jenny Craig, Weight Watchers. What I realized I had to do and will repeat right here at the beginning of this chapter is to clarify that when I refer to the term *diet* I am asking about your daily intake. What do you eat? What types of vegetables do you eat? What color are your carbohydrates? What is your favorite source of sugar?

I do not ask this from a place of judgment, but instead as a source for inspiration. I want to help my clients come up with individualized ways to still enjoy the food they love while effectively contributing to their exercise efforts. Again, keep in mind that any changes are intended to adjust for a lifestyle improvement, not as punishment for a short period of time. These changes should be done in moderation and in gradual increments. The slow evolution of a healthy diet will make it permanent.

BUDGETING CALORIES

As I previously mentioned, I have the worst sweet tooth you will ever see, and I blame it on my parents. My father appreciates sweets as much as I do, and my mother is an excellent cook and provider of all things fabulous. I also believe that I passed this gene onto my son, who loves chocolate with the same passion as his mother. The good news is that I have figured out that you really can be fit and thin and still eat your favorite goodies. Whether you crave the salty snacks or sweet treats, you don't have to give them up to reach your goals.

Nancy was a good four sizes overweight when I met her, partially due to her Cold Stone ice cream addiction. She wanted me to help her comfortably fit into a size six, and she wasn't willing to give up sweets. I have found that it is always possible to reach your goals without eating like someone else. It never works to tell my clients to eat what I eat because they are not me. I can make general suggestions of food items that I like that may work for them, but I can't give them a mandatory menu and expect them to stick to it. It just doesn't work. It is always better to adjust a person's existing behaviors initially, rather than create completely new ones.

I devised a plan for Nancy where she could eat little sweets throughout the day, as long as she stayed within her allotted daily calories. Now, I begged her for months to eat salads and nutrient-dense foods, but she refused. So I monitored her calorie intake and often took home extra goodies that she had baked. I even once agreed to make a cake that she wanted, as long as I only delivered exactly two slices to her. I kept the rest. I'm not sure this plan was working for my waistline, but it did seem to help her! She did her elliptical machine at home on the days we didn't meet, and a year later she was down to her goal weight and a healthy size six. I even talked her into taking a daily multivitamin!

I hope you don't think that I'm suggesting that you live on sweets to lose weight; I'm not! But I am suggesting that you budget your calories enough to enjoy the foods you love. I personally do not get through a day without chocolate or ice cream and sometimes both! Perhaps for you it is chips or bread. Like Nancy, I have learned to budget my calories. I choose to eat light and healthy throughout the day so that I can enjoy that daily chocolate bar without any consequences. I can easily enjoy oatmeal for breakfast and a salad with Ahi tuna for lunch every day, and I can still splurge in the afternoon. Or perhaps I won't eat bread for lunch if I'm having pasta for dinner. It's all about making choices that will fit into your daily budget.

At first you may need to count calories to get an idea of how much you consume. Your goal should be to limit yourself to 1200-1800 calories, depending on how much exercise you are doing. A completely sedentary 150-pound person should eat no less than 1200 calories a day to lose weight. If you are tall or exercise regularly, your caloric goal will be closer to 1600 calories per day. Eventually you won't need to count your calories to know how much you are consuming.

So, how many calories should you be eating in a day? First, you need to determine how many calories your body burns at rest. You may have heard of Resting Metabolic Rate (RMR) and Basal Metabolic Rate (BMR). The difference between the two is that the BMR is often calculated by fasting and then resting whereas the RMR is a calculation of calories based on your ideal weight. The RMR is the amount of calories you burn in a 24-hour period just resting and therefore it represents how many calories you need to consume for your body to perform its regular functions such as breathing, pumping blood and maintaining normal body temperature and organ function. For the purposes of simplicity, we will look at the RMR as a means to determine the amount of calories you should consume to *lose* weight. Let me show you how to figure it out.

HOW MANY CALORIES SHOULD YOU EAT TO LOSE WEIGHT? - CALCULATING RESTING METABOLIC RATE (RMR)

Step 1: Determine your ideal weight.

If you are considerably overweight adjust this number by meeting your ideal weight halfway. For instance, if you are 180 pounds and you were 140 pounds at your healthiest, your ideal weight for this calculation would be 160 pounds. If you are not obese, your ideal weight is just that (140 pounds), what you weighed when you were your healthiest and realistically where you would like to get to as your goal. Set realistic goals. Another common way to calculate your ideal weight is basing it on your height. For men, start with 106 pounds for the first 5 feet, and then add 6 pounds per inch taller than 5 feet. (Ideal weight for a 5' 10" man is 106 + 60 = 166 pounds). For women, start with 100 pounds for the first 5 feet, and then add 5 pounds for each additional inch. (Ideal weight for a 5' 6" woman is 100 + 36 = 136 pounds).

Example: Kathy is tall (5' 9") and weighs 160 pounds. She knows that **her ideal weight is 145 pounds** and she is basing this number on when she was working out consistently, eating well and liked her shape without being too skinny. Or, given her height, her ideal weight is also 145 pounds (100 lbs for the first 5 feet, plus lbs for the additional 9 inches = 145 lbs)

Step 2: Multiply your ideal weight times 10

Example: Kathy's RMR would be 145 (pounds) x 10 = **1,450** calories

This means that she can eat 1,450 calories per day without gaining or losing any weight. But remember that number is what her body burns just breathing and pumping blood. The fact that Kathy works in a busy office and also exercises every other day means she will need to consume more calories to stay healthy.

CALCULATING DAILY CALORIES BURNED FOR WEIGHT LOSS

Step 1: *Add normal daily activity to your RMR.*

If you are active during the day running errands or watching after young children as a single mother, or you work in a busy office and you are often moving from one office to another and attending meetings, you must add on average 50% more calories to your RMR.

Example: Kathy is in charge of operations for her company and she often is walking to and from other departments, training staff and using various office machines not located in her immediate vicinity.

1,450 calories (RMR) x 50% = 725 calories added.

Now Kathy's calories burned per day have increased from 1,450 to **2,175**

Step 2: *Add purposeful exercise to your RMR.*

On the days you go to the gym, take a walk or run, or go for a bike ride, add these burned calories burned to your RMR.

Example: Kathy walks 4 miles, 4 times per week. On those days, she can add the amount of calories she burns from those walks to her daily RMR. Based on her weight and how many minutes it takes her to walk 4 miles (60 minutes or 4 mph), she burned 400 calories or 100 calories per mile. (There are a lot of sites online that can help you find out how many calories you burn during any given exercise.)

2,175 calories + 400 calories = **2,575** calories burned

Example: Kathy has reached a plateau in her weight loss and realizes she needs to add strength training to her regimen a couple of times per week. She takes an intermediate Pilates class and based on her weight, she burns 400 calories per hour.

2,175 calories + 400 calories = 2,575 calories burned

Now Kathy has a better idea of how many calories she can eat on the days she exercises and on the days she does not.

Non-Exercise day	Pilates or Walking Day
1,450 (RMR)	1,450 (RMR)
+ 725 (daily routine)	+ 725 (daily routine)
+ 0 (no purposeful exercise)	+ 400 (walking 4 miles or Pilates class)
2,175 Calories burned per day	2,575 Calories burned per day

As you can see, on the days Kathy does not exercise, she needs to reduce the amount of calories she can consume in order just to maintain her current weight. She can consume either 2,175 calories per day on the non-exercise days, or 2,757 calories on the days *with* exercise. How is that for a reason to work out! She knows that in order to stick to a weight-loss regimen and do it a healthy way, she should be averaging about 1–2 pounds of weight loss per week. To accomplish that she must "bank", or reduce her caloric intact by 500 calories per day. Let me demonstrate.

1 pound is the equivalent of 3,500 calories. Burning 500 more calories per day than is consumed, multiplied by 7 days in a week, equals a 3,500-caloried deficit per week, or the equivalent of 1 pound of weight loss per week.

Example: **Pilates or Walking Day**

2,575 Calories burned

- 500 "Banked" or calorie reduction

2,075 Calories Kathy can eat on that day.

I would NOT advise Kathy to reduce her caloric intact by 1,000 calories per day in order to speed up her weight loss for a couple of reasons. First, that would take her down to 1,175 calories on the days she does not work out which is below her Resting Metabolic Rate and we already determined that she needs 1,450 calories just for her organs to function properly and it will slow down her metabolism. Secondly, reducing to 1,575 calories per day on the exercise days may not provide her enough nutrients to sustain the amount of energy she needs for her exercise and she may get fatigued and possibly sick as a result. Lastly, given her ideal weight and what she currently weighs, losing more than 1 pound per week is not something she can maintain for very long and the way she will have to eat and the lack of energy she will have is not a healthy lifestyle. Mentally and physically it will feel like a grind, a punishment and a diet. This is about maintaining a lifestyle, and not about deprivation.

So be careful not to restrict calories so much that you do not give your body the fuel to burn fat. When you skip meals or don't eat enough before you exercise, you send your body into starvation mode which means it stores fat resulting in burning muscle mass when you exercise. When you consider the fact that muscle burns fat, you want to hold onto as much muscle as possible. So do not deprive yourself of nutrients that your muscles need to work efficiently and *assist you* in your fat-burning efforts.

When you are working out, you can and need to eat healthy, colorful calories. But don't fall into the "I walked 3 miles now I can have that

Frappacino" mentality. Rather than have the mindset that you exercise therefore you can eat, switch it to "I eat therefore I can exercise." See exercise as a positive thing you do for yourself, not a punishment.

CHAPTER SEVEN

THE FOOD FACTOR

"The wise man should consider that health is the greatest of human blessings.
Let food be your medicine."

❖ HIPPOCRATES

WHAT *DO* I EAT?

Now that you know how many calories you can consume per day to maintain or lose weight, you realistically need to know how much you are actually eating. You might think, "Ugh" when I tell you that you should keep a food journal, but hear me out. Just keeping track of what you eat everyday for seven days may be the eye-opener you need to make some changes. Although it may seem tedious, keep in mind that you probably eat the same cereal every morning or prepare the same salad or chicken dish a few times per week. You can find the calorie count of every item either on its package or for fresh, raw items you can look them up online or in a book. There are numerous websites that allow you to either pick from a list of food items and the appropriate quantity and it will calculate the per-serving calories for you. There are also plenty of food calorie counter books on the market that are constantly being updated so that even calories for restaurant meals are listed. Making a list of these dishes and adding up the calories may take a few minutes the first time, but then you never have to do it again because you will have a running list of food items and their calorie count from which to reference. As a guide, below is an abbreviated version of my list.

Item	Quantity	Calories
Whole egg	1 each	75
Egg white	1 each	17
Whole wheat bread	1 slice	90
Almond Butter	1 Tbsp	95
Natural Peanut Butter	1 Tbsp	105
Mixed Greens	3 Cups	20
Fat-Free Milk	1 Cup	90
Tuna – canned, in water	½ can	80

"Eat breakfast like a king, lunch like a prince, and dinner like a pauper."
❧ ADELLE DAVIS (AMERICAN NUTRITIONIST)

WHAT *SHOULD* I EAT?

This seems to be an ongoing battle for many of us. I fit my meals in between clients and I am fortunate that they do not mind the fact that I am just finishing chewing when they arrive for their session. The most common question I get is "what are you eating?" This is not to be nosy, but it is because they, like many of us, are looking for new, creative and delicious ways to fuel our bodies without exceeding our daily calories.

I wanted to take this time to share with you, as I do with my clients, "What Lariesa eats." I believe we are all creatures of habit when it comes to what we purchase, prepare and eat. When I go to the grocery store, I usually end up buying the same staple items and preparing different variations of the same foods. The great thing about this repetition is I

THE FOOD FACTOR   95

no longer have to look up the calories of any food item when I keep track of my daily intake. I now know how much I am eating each day without even writing it down.

Now please keep in mind that I am not a nutritionist nor do I claim to be a self-taught expert on nutrition, but I can tell you what works for me and it may provide you with new ideas. I am also a vegetarian who eats fish. In most cases, my protein choices for lunch and dinner can be replaced with turkey, chicken or beans.

MEAL IDEAS

Breakfast:

Day One	Low sugar oatmeal packet made with hot water and add 2 Tb raisins, or half of a banana
Day Two	Lite N' Fit or nonfat yogurt topped with 1/2 cup bran cereal flakes or whole grain cereal
Day Three	Healthy homemade muffin (see recipe section) plus cantaloupe or fruit
Day Four	1 cup bran oatmeal cereal with 1 cup non-fat milk and a banana, or strawberries and slivered almonds
Day Five	3 scrambled eggs, with only one yolk or hard boiled egg whites plus whole wheat toast and 1Tb jam or peanut butter

I usually pack breakfast to go, and need to eat it at work, so the first three options are a quick and easy way to have breakfast on the run. The other options are when I do not have early appointments or on the weekends.

A note about cereals: They can be the most efficient way to start your day if you eat the right ones. Rather than provide you with a huge list of do's and don'ts, jot down these go-to numbers and check out the cereals currently in your pantry or when you shop for new ones.

Cereal Sense:

Total Fat	3 grams or less
Fiber	5 grams or more
Sugar	8 grams or less
Sodium	250 milligrams or less
Iron	At least 25% Daily Value

THE FOOD FACTOR

Lunch:

Day One	3 cups dark or mixed salad greens with ½ can tuna or ½ a grilled Ahi tuna steak, low-fat or nonfat dressing, or salsa and half an avocado. (You could replace the fish with grilled chicken or beans).
Day Two	Tuna sandwich with nonfat miracle whip or mayo, lettuce, on whole wheat bread (you could replace the tuna with turkey or lean lunch meats).
Day Three	Sandwich wrap with grilled shrimp or fish and veggies, avocado, and veggies such as zucchini, bell peppers, eggplant.
Day Four	Mexican salad made with fresh romaine, black beans, green onions, chopped tomato, a sprinkle of feta cheese, salsa, and 1 Tbnonfat sour cream.
Day Five	3 cups mixed greens, 2 Tblsp chopped unsalted nuts, 1 Tb Feta cheese, ½ can of tuna, low-fat dressing, handful of whole wheat crackers.

Dinner:

Mix and match any of the items below, one from each category.

Lean Protein	Carbohydrate	Vegetables
Salmon	Brown or wild rice	Broccoli, fresh or frozen
Ahi Tuna	Quinoa (also a protein)	Kale or dark greens, spinach
White fish (Halibut, Sea bass)	Couscous	Green beans
Shrimp	Whole wheat bread/roll	Okra
Chicken, grilled or baked	Yams or sweet potato	Mixed vegetables
Lean beef	Small baked potato or red potatoes	Asparagus
Turkey, ground, grilled or baked	Pasta, preferably whole wheat	Zucchini or yellow squash

Snacks:

- Apple, tangerine, banana or other cut fruit such as pineapple or melon

- ¼ cup hummus with ½ whole wheat pita bread or raw veggies

- One slice whole wheat bread with 1 Tbls natural peanut butter

- 1 cup vegetable soup

- Non-fat yogurt with ½ cup strawberries or blueberries

- Sliced apple with 1 Tbls peanut butter

- Banana Bran Muffin (see recipe in back of book)

- A dozen unsalted almonds and a couple of apricots

Healthy Substitutions:

Unhealthy Food Choices	Healthier Substitutes
Fried foods	Bake, broil or grill
Packaged foods (cookies, crackers, potato chips)	Fresh fruit, vegetable, or whole grain and baked chips
Sugary foods (candy bars, ice cream)	Limit quantity or change type (dark chocolate pieces, frozen yogurt with no additions)
Soda, diet or regular (Empty calories that spike blood sugar and make you tired afterwards.)	Try seltzer with a splash of cranberry juice, or Crystal Light.
High-fat condiments (mayonnaise, creamy salad dressings, B-B-Q Sauces, sour cream, cream cheese)	Reduce quantity and/or replace with low-fat or non-fat yogurt
High-fat sauces and soups (anything cream-based – Alfredo, bisques)	Tomato-based or stock soups and marinara sauce
Soft cheeses (cheddar, brie, mozzarella)	Limit consumption to twice per week and portion control. Use a teaspoon of Parmesan or Romano cheeses for flavor to dishes
White pasta or rice	Whole-wheat pasta or brown rice
Iceburg lettuce	Spinach or dark leafy greens
Chicken fingers	Roasted or baked chicken
Hamburger	Turkey or veggie burger

"Strength is the ability to break a chocolate bar into four pieces with your bare hands - and then just eat one of those pieces."

❖ JUDITH VIORST

NOT-SO-INNOCENT SNACKING

We are all guilty of putting stuff into our mouths that we know we shouldn't. It may be the French fries you couldn't resist when your husband stopped at McDonald's, or maybe the handful of chips you grabbed at your last meeting. On most days it may be the bites of food you eat off your kid's plate. Yes, we are all to blame for these daily, yet not-so-innocent bites. The calories add up, and we need to be accountable for them. For example, it is difficult to make healthy food choices when your children's leftover macaroni and cheese is just sitting there. It is too easy to indulge in a few creamy bites over the kitchen sink. I know you've done it because so have I!

It's not easy preparing food and doing laundry, cleaning, working, etc, all at the same time. I have often found myself inhaling my dinner and whatever other snacks (not usually healthy ones) happen to be around. Sitting down to a meal as a single mom never really seemed to happen. I became the all-star multi-tasker, but it wasn't helping my waistline, or my stress level. I have learned to sit at the table with my son, and eat in a way that is calm and better for both of us. It forces you to think about what you are eating, and prevents you from inhaling things unconsciously. Besides, what are we teaching our children when we eat like this?

It almost seems like those not-so-innocent calories don't count if nobody is watching, or if you barely tasted them. Unfortunately, they do count, and they can add up to double-digit pounds. So, how do you avoid these tempting tastes? The easiest way is to let yourself nibble on a stalk of celery while you cook, or a few apple slices. At least you are taking the edge off of your hunger while you prepare food for the family. If you know that you're children's chicken fingers or grilled cheese sandwiches are tempting to you, then give yourself a healthy snack that you can enjoy (maybe not enjoy as much as grilled cheese, but get over it) that will help you avoid picking the leftovers off of their plates.

A good defense is to throw the leftover tempting food right into the trash before you can talk yourself out of it. Just throw it right in and bury it with something else. You know you won't go back for it especially if it's under coffee grinds. I know it seems extravagant, but it works. Even better still, have your children scrape their own plates right into the trash. Not only are you not involved in the fate of the food, but you teach your children a good, helpful routine.

It also works to keep a food diary, or at least write down all of those "mindless" bites. You will be surprised at how many times this happens. You will find it enlightening to see how many calories you consume with this type of snacking. I know you hate to keep a food diary, but it has been proven to work over and over. At least keep the diary for one week to begin to see where the not-so-innocent patterns exist. And don't keep putting it off for a week in which you do not have any dinner plans or outings with your friends. That could be the best time to start, as you will see the potato skins and cocktails add up and you will get a better sense of where you can start shaving off calories.

SNEAKY SOURCES OF SUGAR

It is believed that the average American consumes an average of 5 pounds of sugar per month, or 60 pounds of sugar in a year! Some of the culprits come from unsuspecting foods such as cereal, ketchup, juices and condiments. Low fat foods can be a sneaky source of sugar because manufacturers often add extra sugar to make up for the fat. In the end, it's the calories that count, so you will need to monitor your portion size to avoid weight gain. The more obvious culprits come from the extra cookies, breads and cakes that we love to consume. These foods lead to weight gain, diabetes, and other diseases. So how much sugar should we consume? The smallest possible amount. It is better to get your carbohydrates from complex sources such as whole wheat and grains. Sugar is a simple carbohydrate and is immediately converted to energy, while the rest becomes fat.

There is good news! Consuming only a little less sugar per day can lead to easy weight loss. That leads to my next point:

BEVERAGES MAKE A HUGE DIFFERENCE!

If you drink juice or sodas, read on! You are about to make a huge breakthrough in your weight loss efforts. Most people consume a huge part of their calories in the form of beverages! **A single can of cola is 150 calories, and contains 41 grams of sugar!** Did you know that you could eat **nine** Oreo cookies for the amount of sugar that's in that one can of soda?!!! A Monster energy drink contains 50 grams of sugar, the same amount of sugar as almost eleven Oreo cookies! That should make you think twice before downing that soda! Now don't think that diet soda is the answer either: studies have shown that consuming sugar substitutes may lead to weight gain. Fruit juices may sound healthy, but they are loaded with sugar too. The best idea is to NOT drink these beverages at all. How can a calorie-free beverages and foods pack on the pounds? Read on...

1. Looks are deceiving

Just because the food is sugar-free does not mean that it is calorie-free. People tend to eat more sugar-free or low-sugar foods because they have fewer calories. You end up consuming more calories than if you had a smaller portion of the real thing. It is important to remember that weight loss is a simple equation of calories in versus calories out – it doesn't matter whether the calories come from sugar (carbohydrate), protein or fat. So if you want to lose weight by eating sugar-free foods, including soda, then you have to eat only a small amount.

2. We don't feel satisfied

Foods that don't have sugar, or that are low-sugar, tend to be less satisfying than their regular counterparts. We tend to over indulge in them because they never really satisfy us. It is always better to eat the real thing in small portions than it is to eat the sugar-free variety in large portions. People in Europe do not usually eat "diet" foods the way Americans do, and yet they are much thinner than Americans. This is because they enjoy real food in small portions, rather than over consuming "diet" foods.

3. Sugar cravings get worse

Many experts hypothesize that the sweetness that no-calorie sweeteners give to foods can lead to sugar cravings. This is because sugar substitutes are still very sweet, in fact often sweeter than foods that contain real sugar. Some people crave more sugar after eating sugar substitutes because they were left feeling unsatisfied. This leads to over consumption.

There is a balance to deciding what is going to work best for you. If your morning Splenda in your coffee doesn't send you running to the cookies, then chances are it is a great way to cut out a few calories. Eat foods that contain sugar, either real or no-calorie, in small portions, and you will be successful.

STRESS AND ANXIETY

Stress and anxiety play a huge role when it comes to weight loss. When we are stressed, the body produces the hormone cortisol which causes hunger. Lack of sleep also causes an increase in appetite. This makes us crave foods with white flour, sugar, fat, and salt because they release dopamine and serotonin, which boosts mood. This overeating only fixes the problem temporarily, and leaves us feeling more exhausted and anxious. This stress-overeating cycle is much like consuming drugs or alcohol, and must be overcome by recognizing the behavior, and taking steps to avoid it. Although taking a nap would probably be the best thing, few of us have time for that luxury.

- Try to drink a large glass of water, and eat an apple. It is very difficult to avoid stress eating if you are depriving yourself of calories already.

- Prepare for your most tired and stressful part of your day by going into it with a healthy meal, rather than feeling hungry and ready to eat anything in sight.

- Avoid keeping your favorite stress-eating snacks such as chips and cookies in the house.

- Breathe and relax. Take one thing at a time, recognizing that turning to food will only make you feel worse.

- Realize that it won't go perfectly every day. If one day is a disaster, then prepare to do better the next day. Practice will make next-to-perfect, and it will get easier with practice.

MAKING SMALL CHANGES

George was accustomed to eating high fat foods such as fast food and super-sized options. His mother cooked with grease and butter, and this daily routine was all she knew because that is how her mother cooked. They simply did not know another way to live, nor did another way appeal to them. They did not feel they had the time or willingness to make healthy changes. George came to me after feeling the effects of his high-fat lifestyle. He had high blood pressure, was obese, and had a high risk for heart disease.

Although he wanted to make changes for the better, he simply did not know how. He needed to learn one step at a time, and retrain his way of thinking and taste buds with time. We made small changes slowly by tweaking his diet, and introducing new healthier food options. I taught him how to cook with a light cooking spray instead of butter, and how to order better choices at his favorite fast food restaurants. We began to measure the quantities of calories per cookie, rather than per package. The changes were gradual and permanent. A year later his lifestyle and diet are completely different, yet totally natural to him. He can no longer remember the person he used to be and the choices he used to make. He no longer desires most of the unhealthy foods he used to crave. He has lost a lot of weight and is no longer at a risk for heart disease, nor does he have high blood pressure. Does he say these changes were easy for him? Not at all. Would he be where he is now with fast and abrupt changes to his diet? Not a chance. He would be back where he started.

George was successful because he was patient and consistent with his changes.

- He made only 1 small change per week. For example, he cut out half of the amount of soda that he was drinking, and that's the only change he made for the first two weeks.

- The third week he replaced his morning McDonald's breakfast sandwich for a low-fat yogurt and cereal.

- He changed his Vente Mocha to a smaller size, but didn't cut it out completely.

- By the second month he was avoiding most fried foods, and replaced French fries with a side salad.

- He began to pack a lunch to work, rather than going out for a high-calorie lunch. At the same time he learned to prepare this lunch the night before when he was not rushed.

- He stocked his fridge with cut veggies and washed apples. You won't eat them if they aren't even there! Put fresh fruits and vegetables in the front of the fridge, ready to put into your mouth so that you will grab them first, before anything else. If you see them, you are more likely to eat them.

THE FOOD FACTOR   107

Remember, George made the changes over time, and that is why he is successful today. He learned how to outsmart himself by preparing foods in advance. The trick is the planning.

STRATEGIES FOR LONG-TERM SUCCESS:

- Don't expect every day to be easy and go the way you planned. It won't. Expect there to be pitfalls, and be ready to get right back on track again.

- Plan in advance! You will have a difficult time avoiding pitfalls if you haven't even set yourself up for success.

- Cook a few tuna steaks or chicken breasts during the weekend to eat with salads during the week.

- Stock your cupboard with low-sugar oatmeal packets and non-creamy soups for healthy and quick options.

- Keep frozen vegetables in your freezer for a healthy side that can be quickly warmed in the microwave

- Start to purchase whole wheat bread, and limit your bread intake. ,Be careful when you see a label that reads "Multi-Grain" as that just means there are more than one grain and not necessarily all of them are whole grains. If you have a sandwich for lunch, avoid bread at dinner!

- Stock up on apples and fruit. Cut cantaloupe and keep it in an appealing container on the top shelf of your fridge.

- Keep frozen and individually-sealed fish fillets and chicken breasts in your freezer for a quick and healthy meal, or to cook in advance and take to work.

- Use my trick: if I'm in the mood for juice once in a while, then I fill my cup halfway with juice, and dilute the rest with water. Believe me, you feel like you enjoyed a little, but it doesn't taste good enough to go for more.

- If you have a sweet tooth, try freezing grapes for a sweet refreshing snack.

HIDDEN SABOTEURS

It is always a struggle to lose weight, and it never helps if there are hurdles in front of you that you don't even know exist. For example, I had a client who suddenly stopped seeing results in her weight loss goal. For weeks I tried to figure out what was missing, or going wrong. Was she really going for her walks as she promised she was? Was she cheating in her diet and not telling me about it? She claimed to be doing everything I asked of her and said "I'm going for all of my walks, eating my salad for lunch, healthy meals and snacks, and just one coffee a day". Ah Ha! Stop right there. It seemed so unsuspecting until the light came on in my head. "What kind of coffee?" I asked. After all, we have been through this conversation so many times before. "A Vente Frappacino" she replied. And there you have it. She had no idea that her daily coffee fix packed 800 calories and enough fat to be a substitute for a Big Mac. Her daily coffee was her weight loss saboteur, and she didn't even know it. Now she is saving her waistline and her money at the same time.

This scenario is typical for many of my clients, and it's not even their fault. How are you going to know that your favorite treat is worth half a day's calories if nobody ever told you or you did not do the research by getting the nutritional facts either at the restaurant, online or in a calorie book? Are there unseen hurdles that you have in your daily routine that are sabotaging you? It is amazing how something so small and seemingly insignificant can have such a big effect. Maybe it's time to look deeply into your habits to reveal those saboteurs. Do any of these look familiar to you?

- Fatty snacks or fried and fast foods

- Sedentary lifestyle

- Smoking, drugs, alcohol

- Lack of sleep

- Stressful job

- Not enough water intake

- Social gatherings where food is the focus

- Friends or family who "just want you to be happy"

- Going grocery shopping when you are hungry

- Boredom

I EAT REALLY HEALTHY AND I EXERCISE BUT I AM NOT LOSING WEIGHT!

Usually this comment comes to me with a look on the person's face that they want to blame *me* for their lack of results. I mean, if the diet is so perfect, then it must be a hormonal imbalance or slow thyroid or something. True, but often not the case. I have found that countless times the diet is still to blame. We have covered many sneaky ways that a diet can sabotage all of your good intentions. Let me tell you more.

BEWARE OF HIGH-FAT CONDIMENTS AND FOODS

I mentioned this earlier in my "healthy substitutions" list, but let's make sure it's clear. Going to Subway because that's how Jared lost weight will only backfire if you put mayo on that sandwich. Learn to like mustard if you don't already. It has no fat, but a lot of flavor. Avoid creamy sauces, dressings and condiments. They have a lot of unhealthy fat and calories, and can turn a "healthy" meal into a nightmare. You may think that fresh tomato bisque looks healthy, but think again. It, and many foods like it, are loaded with fat and calories.

IT'S IMPOSSIBLE TO EAT RIGHT AT WORK!

Ok, I have heard it all. You may not have a fridge or a microwave at your disposal at work. Maybe you can't imagine another alternative to the cafeteria. Although you can make healthy choices in your work place cafeteria, it will save you bucks and calories if you pack a lunch. Don't feel shot down. You *can* do this. Look at the list above and get creative about foods that you take to work. The way to make it work is to plan ahead. Keep these foods in your fridge so that they are ready to prepare the night before. At least keep some healthy food from the list that doesn't take preparation so that you can just grab and go. You can make a turkey sandwich and pack it with an apple before you head out. My favorite thing is to cook some tuna steaks or chicken breasts and just keep them in the fridge so that I can just grab them to take to work. Its healthy lean protein, and already done! Perfect. Pair it with a fruit or veggies, and it makes a great "lose weight, but feel no hunger" lunch.

So what if the cafeteria is your only option? Choose a lean meat with veggies and a little complex carbohydrate. That means you should get the salad with chicken (remember, no high-fat Caesar dressing here!). Go ahead and have the hamburger with no bun and extra veggies. A wrap with veggies and turkey or chicken can be healthy if you avoid the dressings. Just get into the habit of avoiding sauces and dressings, and choosing lean proteins with veggies and minimal carbs, and you will be on the right, satiated track.

HOW CAN I AVOID SABOTAGING MYSELF AT A RESTAURANT?

Have you noticed that restaurants are now including the number of calories in the meals? It is a real shocker to find out that an average restaurant entrée has more than 1,000 calories, and that a full salad can pack as many calories as an entrée. So, have you been ordering the Asian salad instead of the chicken pasta in an effort to watch calories? Think again. Most restaurant salads are just as bad as the regular meals. So how do you eat out without eating more than your daily budget allows? It can be done:

- Ask for the "light menu" from the beginning. A lot of restaurants offer healthier menu options, but they may not offer it unless you ask.

- Look at the fat and calories in each of the meals to determine what the reasonable choices are.

- Eat only half. Have the waiter box the second half before he even brings it out to you! If a restaurant meal has 1,200 calories, then eating half would be about right. Take the other half home to look forward to the next day.

- Have any sauces or condiments served on the side. You will slash fat and calories by skipping the hollandaise and gravy.

- Order your meal with two servings of steamed veggies, and leave out the mashed potatoes or rice. You will feel full, and will leave behind hundreds of unwanted fat and calories.

- Eat a small cup of broth based soup or a piece of fruit such as an apple before you get to the restaurant. It will help stay in control and make smart decisions if you aren't famished when you get there. Or start your meal with a light soup, and order a small entrée.

- Did I mention skipping that bread basket? Ok, you already knew. At least limit yourself to one small piece.

THE CARBOHYDRATE CONTROVERSY

Carbs are viewed as the enemy. Why? Because carbohydrates turn into sugar in the body, and we tend to eat too much of them. Here's the problem: if you cut carbs completely out of your diet, then you end up feeling exhausted and miserable, and you end up gaining the weight back in the end. So what's the best way to lose weight that will stay off? Eat a little bit of complex carbs everyday. Let's talk about how to do that. A complex carb is one that is not white or processed. They tend to be dark in color, and have slightly more fiber and nutrients than their simple counterpart. They don't turn to sugar as quickly in the body, and therefore keep you feeling full longer.

Some examples of healthy foods containing complex carbohydrates are:

- Whole Barley

- Buckwheat

- Buckwheat bread

- Oat bran bread

- Oatmeal

- Oat bran cereal

- Muesli

- Wild rice

- Brown rice

- Multi-grain bread

- Pinto beans

- Yogurt, low fat

- Skim milk

- Navy beans

- Yams

- Carrots

- Potatoes

- Soybeans

- Lentils

- Garbanzo beans

- Kidney beans

- Lentils

- Split peas

Some examples of foods containing simple carbohydrates are:

- Bread made with white flour

- Pasta made with white flour

- White rice

- All baked goods made with white flour

- Most packaged cereals

- Soda pop, such as Coke®, Pepsi®, Mountain Dew®, etc.

- Table sugar

- Corn syrup

- Fruit juice

- Candy

- Cake

Learn to choose only complex carbohydrates without looking at the list every time.

Read the labels.

If the label lists sugar, sucrose, fructose, corn syrup, white or "wheat" flour, they contain simple carbohydrates. If these ingredients are at the top of the list, then it is the main ingredient, and should be avoided.

Look for whole foods that are not refined.

It is better to eat the whole fruit than fruit juice, or fresh grapes rather than raisins. Whole grain breads are better than white breads, and so on. Choose oatmeal rather than boxed cereals. Avoid snacks that are in packages and boxes, as they are likely more refined and higher in simple carbs.

What is a serving size of Carbohydrates?

The following is a list of typical serving sizes of common carbohydrates (also referred to as Grains or Starches). Most women need no more than 5 servings of carbohydrates per day when trying to lose weight.

Cereals and Grains:

- 1 oz most cold cereals (1/4 – 1 cup)

- ½ cup cooked cereal (e.g. oatmeal, cream of wheat)

- ½ cup cooked white or brown rice

- ½ cup cooked pasta or Soba noodles

- 3 Tbs wheat germ

Breads:

- 2 slices reduced calorie bread
- ½ hot dog or hamburger bun
- ½ English muffin
- ½ bagel (1 ounce, or about the size of a hockey puck)
- 1 small roll (1 ounce)
- 1 6" diameter corn or flour tortilla

Snack Foods:

- ¾ oz pretzels
- 2 graham crackers
- 4 slices melba toast
- 2-6 baked whole-wheat crackers 6 saltine crackers
- 2, 4" diameter rice or corn cakes

So, if you eat cereal in the morning and a sandwich for lunch, then you have already consumed 3 servings of carbohydrates that day. If you are trying to lose weight, then you should limit your consumption of carbohydrates for dinner, or omit them completely. Load up on lean protein and vegetables to feel full and cut calories. You will also wake up less bloated and ready for a breakfast that contains complex carbohydrates.

THE POWER OF PROTEIN

Now that you know that eating complex carbohydrates are necessary for weight loss and function, it is time to discuss the benefits of eating lean protein. Much has already been stated about fueling up on lean proteins to lose weight, maintain muscle mass, and have radiant skin. However, it is possible to have too much of a good thing, and that will sabotage your weight loss efforts. Eating the right kinds of protein and in the right amount is essential to your health.

Research has found that diets rich in protein can help prevent obesity, osteoporosis, and diabetes. A study at Johns Hopkins University also found that a diet that consists of 25% calories from lean protein sources reduces "bad" cholesterol levels and triglycerides better than a high-carbohydrate diet. Lean protein also acts as an appetite suppressant because it takes longer to leave your stomach, so that you feel fuller sooner, and for a longer amount of time. You also burn more calories digesting and metabolizing lean proteins, which aids in weight loss efforts.

If you are dieting without eating enough lean protein, then up to 50% of the weight you are losing is muscle tissue. This is bad news for anyone trying to look great, because muscle tissue is what helps keep your metabolism revved, and your body toned. If you are working out and limiting calories, then you need to make sure that you are eating enough protein so that the weight you are losing is fat, not muscle. Remember, the more muscle tissue you have, the more calories you burn, even at rest. So it is so important that your body does not metabolize your muscle as fuel!

How much protein should you consume so that you can keep your muscle tissue and still lose weight? Experts advise consuming between 0.8 grams and 1.1 grams of protein per pound of your body weight. That's between 104-143 grams for a 130-pound woman. Aim for the low end if you are trying to lose weight and on the high end if you're very active.

Lean proteins are made up of amino acids which help repair and build muscle tissue. However, not all proteins contain all nine of the amino acids necessary to do this task. The foods that contain all nine amino acids are called complete proteins, and are necessary for supporting biological functions. Foods found in animal products such as eggs, chicken, turkey, seafood, low-fat dairy, lean beef and pork are all complete proteins. It is more difficult to find complete proteins in vegetarian foods, although sources such as soybeans, hempseed, buckwheat and quinoa are considered complete proteins. Aim to fulfill your daily protein requirements with these sources and you are bound to lose weight and keep your metabolism in high gear.

I always start my morning with a complex carb such as oatmeal, or a nonfat yogurt and bran cereal. It gives me a boost of energy and keeps me going for a while. If I eat more carbs for lunch, then I will avoid them for dinner. In other words, if you have a sandwich or wrap for lunch then just eat the lean protein and veggies for dinner, skipping the rice or potatoes. If I want to eat those carbs at dinner time, then I will avoid them at lunch. You will end up eating the right amount of carbs, and you will lose weight without feeling miserable.

Give your body what it needs without excess, and you will lose weight without hating life.

CHAPTER EIGHT

LAREISA'S FAVORITE HEALTHY RECIPES

"To eat is a necessity, but to eat intelligently is an art."

◈ LA ROCHEFOUCAULD

✺ BANANA BRAN MUFFINS

1 egg
¾ cup light brown sugar
1 ½ cups ripe mashed banana
½ cup raisins or walnuts
1/3 cup vegetable or canola oil
1 ½ tsp vanilla extract
¾ cup all purpose flour
¾ cup whole wheat flour
½ cup oat bran
2 tsp baking powder
½ tsp. baking soda
1 tsp ground cinnamon
¼ tsp. salt

Heat oven to 375 degrees. Use baking cups or a light cooking spray. Beat eggs and sugar until smooth. Beat in bananas, raisins, oil, and vanilla. Mix together flours, bran, baking powder, baking soda, cinnamon and salt. Add banana mixture and combine just until moistened.

Scoop batter into muffin cups and bake 15-20 minutes or until brown and springy to the touch.

POPULAR TOMATO APPETIZER

3 beefsteak tomatoes
Queso fresco cheese
Fresh lime juice
Cilantro
Avocado
Salt and pepper

Slice tomatoes ¼ inch thick and arrange on a serving plate. Sprinkle with salt, pepper, and lime juice. Crumble queso fresco and cilantro over tomatoes, and arrange avocado slices on top.

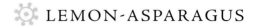 LEMON-ASPARAGUS

1 bunch fresh asparagus
Lemon slices
Olive oil spray

Boil hot water and cook asparagus until crisp-tender. Lightly spray a nonstick skillet with olive oil spray and place asparagus in pan to grill. Toss with lemon juice, salt and pepper.

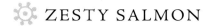 ZESTY SALMON

4 wild salmon steaks
2 Tb. McCormick Montreal chicken seasoning
Fresh lemon slices

Lightly spray a large skillet with cooking spray. Add 4 Tbs water. Place salmon steaks in pan over medium heat. Sprinkle with seasoning, cover, and cook until done. Drizzle with lemon juice and serve with asparagus and brown rice.

BAKED SALMON OVER QUINOA

4 wild salmon steaks
½ cup chopped green onions
½ tsp. crushed red pepper
½ tsp. salt
1 Tb. olive oil
3 Tb. pitted chopped black olives
2 Tb. fresh lemon juice
½ tsp. finely grated lemon zest
1 ½ cups quinoa, rinsed and drained

Preheat oven to 450. In a small bowl, combine green onions, red pepper, salt, and olive oil. Spray a small roasting pan with olive oil spray and arrange salmon in it. Coat the fish evenly with the green onion mixture. Roast the salmon in the top portion of the oven until it is barely opaque, about 15 minutes. Meanwhile, boil 3 cups water in a saucepan. Add quinoa; cover and cook on low heat until the water is absorbed, about 15 minutes. Mix with olives, lemon juice and lemon zest. Serve salmon over quinoa mixture.

LARIESA'S SHRIMP PASTA

1 bag Whole wheat spiral pasta or tri-colored pasta
1 cup cooked shrimp, tail-off
Fresh grated parmesan cheese
1 yellow Onion
3 cloves garlic, minced
¼ cup Olive oil
Garlic powder
Salt and pepper

Boil noodles according to package directions. Set aside. Saute onion and garlic in olive oil until tender. Add shrimp and cook until heated through. Add noodles to onion mixture. Sprinkle with garlic powder, salt and pepper to taste. Sprinkle with parmesan and serve.

✿ MOM'S FAMOUS SPAGHETTI SAUCE

1 yellow onion
8 cloves garlic, minced
½ cup olive oil
1 bunch parsley
4 (14.5oz) cans chopped tomatoes
1 can tomato sauce
1 ½ Tbs. Oregano
1 ½ Tbs. Basil
2 Tbs. honey
1 ½ cups water
1 tsp salt
1 tsp pepper

Sauté the onion and garlic in hot olive oil until translucent and tender. Add the rest of the ingredients and simmer for 1-6 hours. This sauce is excellent the next day.

CHICKEN ENCHILADAS

1 ½ Tb. olive oil
1 medium onion, diced
2 tsp. oregano
Salt and pepper to taste
Flour tortillas
2 chicken breasts, chopped into ½ inch pieces
1 bag frozen stir fry veggies including bell peppers
2 cups shredded Monterey jack cheese
1 jar salsa verde

Heat oil; add onion and sauté until tender. Add chicken and cook until opaque. Add vegetables and oregano and cook until heated through. Season with salt and pepper. Lay out tortillas; divide chicken mixture on each of the tortillas, then roll up and place seam-side down (single layer) on a baking dish covered with cooking spray. Bake at 350 degrees for 25 minutes or until crispy, then cover with shredded cheese and place in oven again for another 10 minutes. Serve with salsa verde, and if desired, chopped olives and tomatoes.

✺ ENERGY COOKIES

1 cup packed brown sugar
2 Tbs. butter, softened
½ cup applesauce
1 large egg
1 cup all-purpose flour
½ cup whole wheat flour
1 ½ cups rolled oats
1 tsp. baking soda
1 tsp. ground cinnamon
¼ tsp pumpkin pie spice
¼ tsp salt
½ cup raisins
½ cup chocolate chips
½ cup white chocolate chips (optional)
1 ½ tsp vanilla

Preheat oven to 350 degrees. Beat sugar and butter until well blended. Add applesauce and egg; beat well. Combine flours, oats, baking soda, cinnamon, pie spice, and salt. Add flour mixture to sugar mixture; beat until well blended. Stir in raisins, chocolate chips, and vanilla. Drop cookies on a baking sheet covered in parchment paper, or cooking spray. Bake at 350 degrees for 10-15 minutes.

ITALIAN LENTIL SOUP

2 carrots, sliced
2 stalks celery, sliced
1 onion, chopped
1 Tb. Olive oil
6 cups water
½ head of cabbage, cored and cut into 1-inch pieces
1 ½ cup dry lentils, rinsed and drained
1 cup tomato puree
1 ½ tsp. sugar
1 ½ tsp salt
½ tsp. dried oregano
¼ tsp. pepper

In a large saucepan cook carrots, celery and onion in hot olive oil about 5 minutes or until crisp-tender. Stir in water, cabbage, lentils, tomato puree, sugar, salt, oregano and pepper. Bring to boiling; reduce heat. Cover and simmer for 45 minutes or until lentils are very soft. Makes 5 servings.

PASTA WITH BASIL AND SPINACH

Penne pasta
Tomatoes, chopped
Bell pepper, chopped
Basil, chopped
Parsley, chopped
Spinach, chopped
Garlic, minced
Olive oil
Salt and pepper
Fresh grated parmesan

Cook pasta. Add all other ingredients in another bowl and let sit it olive oil, garlic, and salt and pepper. Add to pasta when finished, top with a generous portion of parmesan.

WHOLE GRAIN SPAGHETTI WITH BELL PEPPERS

12 ounces whole-wheat or spelt spaghetti
1 ½ Tb. Olive oil
½ red onion, chopped
4 bell peppers (one each green, red, orange, yellow), cored and chopped
½ jalapeno, seeded and minced (optional)
3 tsp. red wine vinegar
¼ cup grated parmesan cheese
Black pepper

Cook spaghetti according to package directions. Sauté onion in olive oil in a medium skillet. Add the bell peppers and jalapeno. Cook until the peppers are soft, about 12 minutes, then stir in red wine vinegar. Toss the pepper mixture with the cooked spaghetti and top with grated parmesan.

VEGGIE GREEK SALAD WITH CHICKPEAS

½ cucumber, diced
2 tomatoes, chopped
1 red bell pepper, chopped
1 green pepper, chopped
½ red onion, thinly sliced
¼ cup chopped black olives
4 Tb red wine vinegar
Crumbled feta cheese

Mix all ingredients and toss with red wine vinegar. Sprinkle with feta cheese and serve with a light ranch dressing, if desired.

ABOUT THE AUTHOR

LARIESA BERNICK has been in the fitness industry for more than a decade. She started out as a certified aerobics instructor and eventually became a personal trainer. She opened her own personal training business, but when her back went out, she turned her focus to Pilates. Pilates was the jumpstart to a new career and a healthy back. She became certified by Balanced Body University and put a single reformer in her garage. Soon Lariesa's clients were as passionate about the benefits of Pilates as she was. It didn't take long for Lariesa to open a complete Pilates studio, Pilates of Eastlake, in California, which has grown with record speed. Lariesa is genuinely dedicated to making a difference in the lives of others by helping reach their goal.

Personal Trainer- ACE
Pilates Instructor- BBU
Group Fitness Instructor- ACE
Weight Management Consultant- ACE
Absolute Body Power Show, Comcast cable TV
Miss Teen Washington State

Basics II Pilates DVD
Basics II Yoga DVD
Basics II Strength DVD

Pilates of East Lake
www.PilatesofEastLake.com

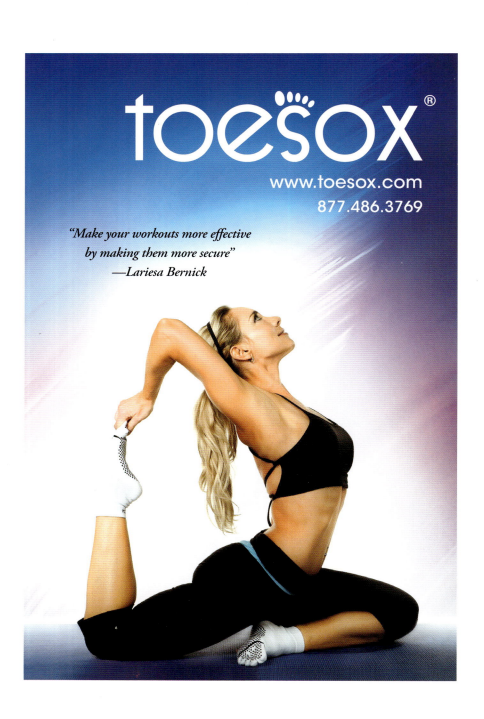